T0146034

UNDER THE BIG TREE

UNDER THE BIG TREE

Extraordinary Stories from the Movement
to End Neglected Tropical Diseases

Ellen Agler with Mojie Crigler

FOREWORD BY BILL GATES

 Johns Hopkins University Press   Baltimore

Johns Hopkins University Press
2715 North Charles Street
Baltimore, Maryland 21218-4363
www.press.jhu.edu

Library of Congress Cataloging-in-Publication Data

Names: Agler, Ellen, 1972– author. | Crigler, Mojie, 1972– author.
Title: Under the big tree : extraordinary stories from the movement to end
     neglected tropical diseases / Ellen Agler with Mojie Crigler ; foreword by
     Bill Gates
Description: Baltimore : Johns Hopkins University Press, 2019. | Includes
     bibliographical references and index.
Identifiers: LCCN 2018020737 | ISBN 9781421427232 (hardcover : alk. paper) |
     ISBN 1421427230 (hardcover : alk. paper) | ISBN 9781421427249 (electronic)
     | ISBN 1421427249 (electronic)
Subjects: | MESH: Neglected Diseases—prevention & control | Tropical Medi-
     cine | International Cooperation | Disease Eradication | Africa
Classification: LCC RC961 | NLM WC 680 | DDC 362.1969/883—dc23
     LC record available at https://lccn.loc.gov/2018020737

A catalog record for this book is available from the British Library.

One hundred percent of author proceeds from this book will be donated to
programs combating neglected tropical diseases.

*Special discounts are available for bulk purchases of this book. For more informa-
tion, please contact Special Sales at 410-516-6936 or specialsales@press.jhu.edu.*

Johns Hopkins University Press uses environmentally friendly book materi-
als, including recycled text paper that is composed of at least 30 percent
post-consumer waste, whenever possible.

CONTENTS

Photographs appear following page 86

Imagine a mosquito biting you. It's infected with tiny larvae, which enter your body and set up camp in one of your lymph nodes. They mate and nest, causing your leg to eventually swell to ten times its usual size.

Left untreated, this painful and disfiguring disease, known as lymphatic filariasis (LF), can lead to permanent disability and social stigma. And it is only one of twenty neglected tropical diseases (NTDs) that afflict more than a billion people, mainly in the developing world.

Spread by worms, insects, and bacteria, NTDs cause immense human suffering. In the worst cases, they kill. And all of them can be prevented—if the world continues to work together to end them.

I recently had the opportunity to join a group of health workers in a rural village in Tanzania who were going door to door to distribute medicines to help eliminate LF. Their passion and tireless efforts were inspiring because they're helping break the cycle of transmission to finally end this terrible disease.

In 2012, 1.5 billion people needed preventive drug treatment to protect them from LF. Since then, thanks to the work of health workers like those I met in Tanzania, LF has been eliminated in eleven countries and reduced in many others.

My wife, Melinda, and I have been proud to be part of the global effort to beat NTDs. In 2012, our foundation joined a coalition of pharmaceutical companies, governments, health organizations, and charities that made a commitment to controlling and eliminating ten NTDs.

The progress has been amazing. In 2016 alone, more than 1 billion people were reached with NTD treatments.

Still, there's a lot of work to be done. We need additional support from the public and from philanthropic sectors in order to reach more people who need treatment. We need better drugs and diagnostics to treat people more quickly and effectively. And we need to continue supporting frontline health workers so they can help more people, especially in hard-to-reach areas.

Under the Big Tree shines a spotlight on some of the heroes in the ambitious effort to rid the world of NTDs. Their stories are an inspiration and, I hope, a rallying cry for others to join the global efforts to finally end the suffering caused by these ancient diseases.

I'm optimistic that together we can lift the burden of these preventable diseases and improve the lives of millions of people around the world.

Bill Gates

APF: African Philanthropy Forum

APOC: African Programme for Onchocerciasis Control

CDC: Centers for Disease Control and Prevention

CDD: community drug distributor or community-directed distributor

CDTI: community-directed treatment with ivermectin

DALYs: disability-adjusted life years

DEC: diethylcarbamazine

DFID: Department for International Development (United Kingdom)

DRC: Democratic Republic of the Congo

ESPEN: Expanded Special Project for Elimination of NTDs

GTMP: Global Trachoma Mapping Project

HKI: Helen Keller International

IOCC: International Orthodox Christian Charities

ITI: International Trachoma Initiative

KEMRI: Kenya Medical Research Institute

LF: lymphatic filariasis

MDA: mass drug administration

MDG: Millennium Development Goal

MDP: Mectizan Donation Program

MoHCC: Ministry of Health and Child Care (Zimbabwe)

MSD: Merck Sharp & Dohme

NatPharm: National Pharmacy (Zimbabwe)

NGDO: nongovernmental development organization

NGO: nongovernmental organization

NTD: neglected tropical disease

OCP: Onchocerciasis Control Program

PCD: Partnership for Child Development

RSC: Rockefeller Sanitary Commission

SAFE: surgery, antibiotics, facial cleanliness, and environmental improvement

SCI: Schistosomiasis Control Initiative

STH: soil-transmitted helminth

TT: trachomatous trichiasis

UN: United Nations

USAID: United States Agency for International Development

WHO: World Health Organization

Nearly two dozen diseases have been designated "neglected tropical diseases." The most prevalent are river blindness, trachoma, lymphatic filariasis, schistosomiasis, and intestinal worms (roundworm, whipworm, and hookworm). These five NTDs are the focus of this book.

NTDs exist in at least 149 countries. This book concentrates mainly on countries in Africa, which shoulders the heaviest burden.

In today's big, bold effort to end NTDs can be found many heroes and many inspiring stories.

Here are a few of them.

CHAPTER ONE

Crisis and Collaboration

On the second day of a conference in 2012, Dr. Massitan Dembélé took the lectern. Her fellow presenters in the main ballroom of La Palm Royal Beach Hotel in Accra, Ghana, were several dozen neglected tropical disease (NTD) program managers from countries throughout Africa. These men and women directed their governments' efforts to treat, prevent, and, in many cases, eliminate a group of parasitic and bacterial afflictions that, although they affect more than 1.5 billion people worldwide, have historically been greatly ignored.

Turned-in eyelashes that scratch the cornea, relentless itching due to millions of worms in the skin, blindness, bloody urine, enlarged scrotums, elephantine legs and feet, not to mention anemia, malnutrition, stunted growth, stunted cognitive development, and increased risk for complications from diseases such as HIV/AIDS— these are but a few sequelae of various NTDs, whose sufferers often drop out of school and live on the margins of society, sometimes stigmatized and abandoned by their families. NTDs are both a source and a result of poverty. The 1.5 billion people who suffer from them are among the poorest in the world.

One after another, the program managers reported on disease prevalence, funding gaps, and current concerns. "Smartphones would help us better share data," said one. "A single vehicle for our entire program isn't enough to reach the remote villages," said another.

Two months into my job as the CEO of the END Fund, I had come to the conference to listen and learn. The END Fund itself was a newcomer to the space, founded in early 2012 by the Dubai-based private investment firm Legatum and its philanthropic advisor, Geneva Global. Back in 2006, one of Legatum's principals had read a *Financial Times* article that quoted a scientist who said that most NTDs "do not need innovation but simply modest funding and a little imagination." Fifty cents per person per treatment, on average, is the cost to treat and prevent the most common NTDs. The price is so low thanks largely to pharmaceutical companies that donate drugs worth billions of dollars. But even more expensive procedures—for example, surgeries to prevent trachoma-caused blindness—cost at most about $100. Changes in hygiene practices, which contribute to preventing some NTDs, cost nominal amounts for training educators, creating informational material, and generating outreach through radio and other media.

The great impact for such a small price was crystal clear to Legatum, which sought to bring an investor's strategic mind-set to the NTD challenge. In April 2012, I was the END Fund's first full-time hire.

Now it was June, and Dr. Dembélé, the NTD program manager for Mali, stood before the crowd. In addition to the NTD program managers, there were nongovernmental organizations (NGOs) that supported the national programs, the major donors that helped pay for them, drug-donating pharmaceutical companies, policy makers, and representatives from the countries' Ministries of Health.

"I would love to tell you how successful our program is," said Dembélé. "But we're in crisis."

With one of the first large-scale programs to integrate NTD treatments, Mali had been heralded as a spectacular triumph, a model for other countries. In 2011, more than 20,000 trained community health workers had treated more than 11 million people concurrently for intestinal worms, lymphatic filariasis (LF), on-chocerciasis (onko-ser-KY-ah-sis, aka river blindness), schistoso-miasis (shisto-so-MY-ah-sis, aka bilharzia), and trachoma. Men and women, young and old, are disfigured and debilitated by these diseases, through blindness (in the case of river blindness and trachoma); grossly enlarged legs and genitalia (LF); itching some-times severe enough to cause suicide (river blindness); or anemia, undernutrition, and growth stunting (schistosomiasis and intesti-nal worms). Moreover, most people with one NTD usually have another NTD. For example, their bodies may be under siege from parasitic worms lodged in their intestine, which are robbing them of nutrients, while *another* kind of parasitic worm causes blood loss from the lining of their bladder. To treat and prevent these diseases is to help communities prosper. More children attend school, more adults work. Productivity rises. Fewer people are shunned by society. Fewer people needlessly die.

Only five years before this conference, these NTDs were being handled by separate, underfunded programs within Mali's Min-istry of Health, with sporadic distributions of medicine occur-ring at different times throughout the year, if at all. By integrating the NTD program, injecting some capital through a grant by the United States Agency for International Development (USAID), and enlisting experts from Helen Keller International (HKI), In-ternational Trachoma Initiative (ITI), and Schistosomiasis Control Initiative (SCI), Mali had drastically reduced not only the number of cases, but the cost of treatment.

Then, in late March 2012, soldiers in the Mali military had staged a coup d'état, overthrowing the government, sending the president into exile, and putting a military junta in power. Amid a slew of international sanctions, the United States had suspended all nonemergency humanitarian aid to Mali. Without the USAID money, the integrated NTD program could not continue.

Dr. Dembélé was the force behind the program. A bureaucratic samurai, working quickly and efficiently within the government to turn an extraordinary number of ideas into action, Dembélé never stopped advocating on a personal level. She knew people's names, where they lived, their disease histories, their families. For people with advanced elephantiasis she had helped create a support and physical therapy group, a novel concept in Mali. She trekked to isolated regions of the country to ensure that the right medicines were delivered on time to the people most in need.

Now she stood before us panicking. It had taken five years to scale the integrated program. In other words, she and her staff had spent five years

- training local health workers on dosage and medical record keeping;
- coordinating the Ministries of Health, Finance, and Education, as well as the donors giving financial support and the local and international NGOs providing on-the-ground and technical support;
- creating and handing out pamphlets and other literature explaining disease transmission and treatment;
- lining up radio stations to play catchy NTD infomercials;
- training DJs to talk about the diseases, both to normalize treatment and so people knew when community health workers were coming to their village;
- and mapping the diseases, that is, tracking where the NTDs were in a country twice the size of Texas with poor and remote rural areas (which had the highest prevalence of NTDs).

The year 2012 was supposed to be a year of full national coverage.

Most heartbreaking was knowing that the diseases' prevalence, which had started to drop, might rise again. At least five to seven years of annual treatment are necessary to break the transmission cycle of LF, for example, to start reining in the disease so it no longer poses a significant public health threat. Mali was just crossing that threshold. A single year without treatment could be a golden opportunity for the disease to resurge. The next mass drug administration (MDA)—when medicine would be distributed throughout Mali—was scheduled for October.

Dembélé wasn't the only one panicking. Mali was an important initiative for private donors (e.g., the Conrad N. Hilton Foundation) and NGOs (e.g., The Carter Center and Sightsavers). HKI, working with Mali's Ministry of Health, had led the integrated NTD treatment effort. But having little unrestricted funding, HKI couldn't cover the financial gap.

Mozambique, Angola, the Central African Republic—these countries, with high NTD burdens and little money for treatment, already had been set as the END Fund's priorities. Mali was not on our list. Nevertheless, through the remainder of the conference, I returned again and again to what I had heard from Dembélé, HKI, and USAID, whose Angela Weaver said to me, "You're working on funding. Do you think you could help?" Warren Lancaster, a senior vice president at the END Fund, was encouraging: "We might really make a difference here." A little more than a million dollars would ensure that the October MDA could go forward.

I was thinking three things:

1. *Disasters can be more compelling for fundraising*. More compelling, that is, relative to programs that address ongoing, entrenched problems. Donations pour in after a disaster because people are suffering acutely *now*, and the event often captures the attention of the media and general public. Waiting may mean a donation comes too late. Based on my experience fundraising in the aftermath of the 2010 earthquake in Haiti (when I worked for Operation Smile) and in Indonesia after the 2004 tsunami (when I was with

International Medical Corps), I knew that NGOs could mobilize emergency funds relatively quickly. Mali was in crisis; I should be able to raise some money to help.

2. *Here's a chance to show value.* The END Fund was new to the field. People didn't know us. Some were skeptical of what we were trying to do. We were still proving ourselves. I was still proving myself. I was hungry to make something work.

3. *Walk the walk.* The concept of servant leadership had been a significant part of my early discussions with Legatum. How could the END Fund best serve the NTD cause? How should we respond to the needs of the community? How could we build something that would be of service to the collective movement? Dembélé had issued a loud, urgent call for help. Mali was a clear priority. If we didn't respond, we were not living up to our values.

A month later, I sat in a conference room in San Francisco's Four Seasons Hotel, facing three of Legatum's senior members. Still in the critical first ninety days of my job, I was there to present a strategic plan and a way forward for the END Fund. While I'd had some preliminary conversations about Mali with Legatum partner Alan McCormick, my vision had been to explain the situation and announce that I had already raised the money. So far, however, I had only one donor.

A hundred people and organizations had turned me down. They couldn't provide the money that fast. NTDs were not their priority. They only funded programs exclusively treating children. They only funded programs *not* treating children. The request didn't fit into their funding cycle. There were a hundred ways to say no, and I heard them all. But whenever someone declined, I asked for the name and number of another potential lead. One such recommendation came from the Children's Investment Fund Foundation and led to my sole donor, Vitol, an oil and gas company that had recently acquired Shell in Mali. The morning of my meeting with Legatum, I had received a message that the Vitol Foundation, the company's philanthropic arm, would contribute $100,000, which was fantastic—but not enough.

The fortune behind Legatum had been made from bold investments in uncharted, frontier markets, including Hong Kong real estate in the 1980s, Brazilian telecommunications in the 1990s, post-Communist Russia, and Japan in the banking crisis of the mid-2000s. I wanted to demonstrate that I deserved a place at this table. Yet here I was, presenting a plan for a country that wasn't on the END Fund's initial priority list and admitting that I'd raised only 10 percent of the funds needed.

"Our investment experience had taught us that opportunity always arises at the most inconvenient moments," Christopher Chandler, Legatum's founder, later recalled. The budget for the Legatum Foundation, the company's philanthropic division, was already fully committed, but the urgency of the situation was evident. The Legatum partners were quick to see the situation through a lens common to investment banking: they offered to underwrite the cost of the program for the coming year, but on the condition that I "syndicate the deal" to other investors. Their willingness to fund any shortfall, up to the cost of the entire program if necessary, enabled me to give Dembélé confirmation that the program could continue and bought me time to find other sources. Drug procurement and health worker training could move forward on schedule as I continued to hustle.

As a fundraiser, I had always partnered with companies local to the cause. When I worked with Operation Smile in Bogotá, we received funding from a steel company, the coffee growers association, and local representatives of multinational companies like Colgate Palmolive and Johnson & Johnson. This approach was universally beneficial. People helped their communities. Companies gained recognition for their civic engagement. A broad spectrum of the population learned about an issue. When I was looking for donors for Mali, however, I didn't have a refined outreach strategy—there wasn't time to develop one, plus I was too green in the field—so I was simply calling every potentially helpful person and organization I knew. That included nontraditional donors, such as the oil and gas company Vitol, which made that first crucial donation.

At the time, gold mining made up a whopping 20 percent of the economy in Mali, which was the third largest gold producer in Africa. Mining companies built schools and health clinics in their particular regions, but they hadn't often partnered with each other or taken on projects at a national level. But Mark Bristow, the CEO of Randgold, Mali's largest gold mining company, liked our pitch. A healthy Mali was in the miners' best interest. Plus, this was great public relations. Bristow volunteered to solicit the other mining companies to join Randgold. A joint effort would bring in more funds and spark media interest. Soon, AngloGold Ashanti, IAMGOLD, Gold Fields, and others were on board. Mining companies had been significant investors in public health causes in Africa, including fights against malaria and HIV/AIDS. Now they could play a role in NTDs. Mark Bristow turned out to be a champion for the cause, bringing his community together to contribute more than $750,000, the bulk of what was needed.

New not only to Mali and NTDs but as an organization was the Margaret A. Cargill Foundation. I approached MACF (which has since been restructured as Margaret A. Cargill Philanthropies) because it was still designing its strategy, looking at potential investments, and giving out initial grants. Margaret A. Cargill, the granddaughter of the founder of agricultural giant Cargill, Inc., had arranged that when she died, her shares in the company would be converted into a foundation and given away. Her death in 2006 created an institution worth more than $5 billion, one of the biggest American foundations. MACF covered the remaining funding gap in Mali.

"The Ministry of Health and its partners are organizing a mass treatment campaign against oncho, intestinal worms, and bilharzia starting October 31, 2012, in the regions of Kayes, Koulikoro, Sikasso, Ségou, and Mopti," said the radio announcement—in English, Bambara, Sénoufo, Fulfulde, Songhoi, Maure, and Dogon. "Via community radio stations, relays, and public announcers, each district will announce its schedule and the kinds of drugs that will be distributed."

A message from HKI was also broadcast:

> They are bad diseases, which may cause poverty while altering your health. Bilharzia may cause nonreversible complications. A lot of blindness cases are attributed to oncho. Intestinal worms cause anemia, while there are a lot of very efficient medications against these diseases. During this distribution campaign, the drugs will be given for free to people who are 5 years old and beyond. To succeed, all the people who are concerned have to be treated and anyone who does not take these drugs becomes a danger for others. Let's mobilize to take these drugs during the campaign. Let's not forget to eat before taking the drugs against bilharzia.

In Kalabankoro, Mali, I watched as a large crowd gathered for the launch of the campaign. The griot—a traditional leader who combines the roles of storyteller, musician, arbitrator, and poet—explained to the crowd where the medicine came from, what it would do, and why they should take it. Hundreds of villagers gathered to listen, then watched as the griot took the pills. The village chief took the pills. The head of police took the pills. They were demonstrating that the drugs were safe. They were saying, "We are doing this together." Music started up—men on drums, women singing, children pounding their feet in traditional dance—and jubilant villagers formed a line, one by one standing next to the height-and-dose pole, then taking the appropriate number of pills. They put me in the line, and I took some pills too. In total that year, throughout the country, approximately 20,000 community health workers treated close to 10 million Malians.

■   ■   ■

This is not a story about raising money. It's about the partnership forged by local and international organizations, from both the private and public sectors, that shared the same goal: to see Mali unencumbered by NTDs. The funding came together because of the dedication of people already involved in the program and the willingness of newcomers to take action quickly and substantially.

USAID is not designed to be flexible in quickly reallocating funds. Government rules and regulations are strongly defined and subject to a diplomatic agenda. Moreover, Mali's NTD program was one of dozens in jeopardy following the coup. It couldn't receive all of USAID's attention. As a private philanthropic group, however, the END Fund could move swiftly and nimbly among many partners. Ultimately we raised close to $2 million, which covered Mali's NTD program for two years, at which point, with a democratically elected president back in power, USAID resumed its funding.

Two million dollars is not, in the grand scheme of things, a lot of money. The cost to remove NTDs from people's lives is a crumb in the context of global health funding; it is estimated that less than 1 percent of global health funding goes to this work. But the impact on individual lives is enormous—either way. Does this child drop out of school to lead his blind elder around the village, or does he stay in school, grow up healthy, find a good job, and contribute to his community? Does this woman's schistosomiasis develop into fatal bladder cancer, or does she raise her children, cook the family's meals, and add to her family's income by selling some of their vegetables at the market? Not only are NTDs relatively inexpensive to treat and prevent, but their absence yields a sizable return. Every dollar spent on NTD prevention is estimated to turn into more than $50 in productivity. Achievement of the control and elimination targets set by the World Health Organization (WHO) would generate US$229 billion in productivity by 2030, according to an Erasmus University study by William K. Redekop and colleagues, published in 2017.

The bedrock of Mali's 2012 triumph was its aggressive, calculated program, which had raised treatment coverage and lowered costs. Because time and resources had been given to mapping the country, Mali was treating specific diseases only where they were endemic; diseases that weren't in a particular region weren't treated there. Follow-up surveys offered proof that the program was effective. You could say that the program, though robust, remained vulnerable to unstable national politics. Or you could say that the program survived *despite* the coup.

Success in Mali was possible. It could be done, and it was. The same is true of many other NTD milestones in recent years. As of early 2018, trachoma has been eliminated in seven countries, and lymphatic filariasis has been eliminated in eleven countries. River blindness, once endemic in multiple foci in Latin America, today lingers in the Americas only in the most remote jungles on the border of Brazil and Venezuela.*

Colloquially, the words "control," "eliminate," and "eradicate" are often interchanged. In public health, though, they represent

---

*As of June 2018, WHO has validated the elimination of trachoma as a public health problem in Cambodia, Ghana, Lao PDR, Mexico, Morocco, Nepal, and Oman; validated the elimination of LF as a public health problem in Cambodia, Cook Islands, Egypt, Maldives, Marshall Islands, Niue, Thailand, Togo, Tonga, Sri Lanka, and Vanuatu; and verified the elimination of onchocerciasis in Colombia, Ecuador, Guatemala, and Mexico.

quite different goals. In general, to "control" a disease is to bring its prevalence below a certain level, even if ongoing preventive treatment is needed. To "eliminate" or "eliminate as a public health problem" means the disease prevalence is so low that mass treatment is no longer needed and the disease no longer represents a significant threat to public health. "Elimination" can also mean that so little of the disease is circulating between humans and vectors that, effectively, the cycle of transmission has been interrupted. To "eradicate" a disease is to end it completely, to have zero known cases. Smallpox remains the only human disease that has been declared eradicated.

The nuances in the definitions of disease control, elimination, and eradication can lead to confusion among the general public. Even among global health professionals, there are ongoing debates and continuing efforts to refine the definitions and guidelines for each disease. Global health leader Dr. William H. Foege told me that even though smallpox was officially declared eradicated in 1980—and there has not been a single case since—there remains a very small group of people who object to its classification as eradicated. They point out that the disease still exists in laboratories in the United States and Russia, and they argue that the "eradication" definition should be extended to include the destruction of lab samples.

Despite the complexities of disease end goal definitions, the vision of a world safe from NTDs is not a pipe dream. In many places, it has been accomplished. Partnerships, funding, strategic programs, and the belief that it can be done—these are the keys to ending these horrific diseases.

In the fifth century BCE, Hippocrates described roundworm. A statue of Egyptian pharaoh Mentuhotep II from 2000 BCE shows swollen legs typical of elephantiasis, which is caused by LF. The Ebers papyrus from 1550 BCE includes treatments for trachoma.

Much of the very long history of NTDs is a list of symptoms and treatments, some torturous. Then, between the 1850s and the early twentieth century, scientists began identifying the parasites and bacteria that cause the diseases, uncovering their life cycles and tracking their means of transmission. The decades following World War II saw a boom in medical progress, including increased attention to impoverished people and these "great neglected diseases," as the late Ken Warren of the Rockefeller Foundation called them. Drug donations from pharmaceutical companies, funding from major foundations and the US and UK governments, and the integration of once-separate disease programs all have contributed to a swell of awareness, a realization that the goal of lifting this burden is "not a million miles away," as Dr. Anthony Solomon at WHO put it. With much success behind us, and more work to do, we are at a tipping point for NTDs.

What will the future be?

It could be this:

These diseases plagued humans for thousands of years. Then, following radical advancements in medicine, technology, and global collaboration, they didn't.

CHAPTER TWO

Modern Approaches to Ancient Diseases

The treatment room had no examination table, no charts on its peach and white walls, no panes in the single window, no electricity, no running water. On the smooth cement floor on a teal woven blanket lay Nieba. At her head was seated an ophthalmic nurse, his back against one wall, legs extended on either side of his elderly patient. He washed her face with orange-brown Betadine disinfectant, patted her dry, then covered her face with a linen cloth into which a small hole had been cut, leaving only her right eye visible.

In the village of N'Gara in western Mali, Nieba was going blind. Trachoma, the result of numerous *Chlamydia trachomatis* infections, had inflamed and warped the skin on the underside of Nieba's eyelid, pulling her eyelashes inward so they scraped her cornea. It's "like sand scratching your eyeball every time you blink," one woman told me. The unrelenting pain drives many people to pluck out their eyelashes. This advanced stage of trachoma, called trachomatous trichiasis (TT), usually precedes corneal opacity and permanent blindness.

Nieba lay on the floor, her face—her identity—covered, except for that eye, which was the demarcation between two lives. Without sight, could she continue to farm, cook, and sell her vegetables at the weekly village market? How would her role in her family change? How would her family change? Nieba's greatest concern, she'd told me that morning, was that if she were blind she would not be useful. Being a burden on others was a worse prospect than the constant pain and severe sensitivity to light she now experienced.

Trachoma spreads by contact with contaminated people and by flies that carry *Chlamydia trachomatis* bacteria from one person to the next. Eye discharges attract the flies, as do human feces. Places with endemic trachoma—rural parts of Africa, Asia, the Middle East, the Pacific islands, and Latin America—have several common features: overcrowded dwellings, little or no clean water or sewage disposal, and, typically, a dry, dusty landscape (though in recent years, severe trachoma has been found in several populations in the Amazon region). Children are most likely to be affected; as the primary caregivers, women are three times more likely than men to develop TT. A person usually needs more than 150 *C. trachomatis* infections to reach TT; in other words, people with TT have basically lived with an ongoing eye infection throughout their lives.

Sightsavers, a UK-based NGO, was underwriting Nieba's surgery, one of thousands it organized and paid for in 2012. Almost immediately upon meeting me, Caroline Harper, the CEO of Sightsavers, had insisted I witness a trachoma surgery. "You'll never forget it," she'd said, and put me in touch with a local team, which had brought me to N'Gara and Nieba.

The simplicity of the undertaking was remarkable. The nurse was in effect a mobile surgical unit, riding his motorbike on unpaved roads to operate on people who could not reach a medical clinic. Working with an assistant, he sometimes performed more than twenty procedures in a day. I'd watched as he'd taken from his satchel his surgical equipment and his lunch. The treatment room was bare but for the blanket Nieba lay on. During my time working at Operation Smile, I had watched numerous surgeries, mostly craniofacial and cleft lip and palate reconstruction, but they were always in a completely sterile environment—the practitioners wore not just gloves, which Nieba's surgical nurse also wore, but masks and gowns. "Surgery" meant a designated operating room in a hospital or clinic, usually with electricity, running water, anesthesia, and surgical equipment. Dr. Anthony Solomon, a medical officer in WHO's Department of Control of Neglected Tropical Diseases, told me that he first saw a TT surgery "on the veranda of a schoolhouse." But, he added, "it makes sense. The eyelid is very vascular. Your risk of having infection is very limited. It's quite a quick procedure. That also limits your risk of infection. Really, you need good lighting and a surgeon who's well trained, with a good steady hand."

Egyptians in the sixteenth century BCE scraped the eyelid to turn the eyelashes away from the eyeball, pulled out the lashes, and/or applied various mixtures of myrrh, urine, lizard dung, and the blood of donkeys, bats, pigs, and goats. In the first century CE, Romans rubbed infected eyelids with red-hot iron needles to cauterize the roots of inward-turning eyelashes. In 2012, Nieba's surgery began with anesthetic drops in her eye, followed by several injections of lidocaine to numb her eyelid.

The nurse placed two hemostats—blood-stanching clamps—onto Nieba's eyelid, a few millimeters in from either end. He cut the skin and muscle just above the edge of the lid, running the incision between the hemostats, careful not to cut all the way through. Then he flipped the eyelid and cut the skin and muscle underneath. Into the incision he inserted a closed pair of scissors, pushing until the scissors emerged through the top of the eyelid. Then he opened the scissors so their blunt sides spread apart any remaining intact muscle. The hemostats were removed and blood flowed profusely, which the nurse dabbed with squares of surgical gauze. Then, with three sutures, he reattached the lower portion of Nieba's eyelid to the upper portion, tying the knots firmly so the eyelashes pointed well away from the cornea. The nurse cleaned and bandaged Nieba's eye, then sent her home. This surgery, which had been performed without electricity and without even a table in the room, had taken twenty minutes and cost about $86.

By altering the angle of Nieba's eyelashes, the surgery had altered her life. Not only was she spared excruciating pain, but she could return to her work and family without the fear of going blind. None of her grandchildren would be obliged to drop out of school to care for her or shoulder her household responsibilities. Like many treatments for trachoma—and other NTDs—the TT surgery is simple and inexpensive, with benefits that reach far beyond the patient herself.

■ ■ ■

In 1999, after studying at the London School of Hygiene & Tropical Medicine, Dr. Solomon had joined his professor, the longtime trachoma advocate Dr. Allen Foster, in helping the Ghana Health Service repurpose its successful Guinea worm program for trachoma. (By 2017, Guinea worm—which is on WHO's list of recognized NTDs—was reduced from several million known cases per year to a mere *thirty* worldwide.) Ghana was one of five pilot countries receiving the antibiotic azithromycin from the International Trachoma Initiative (ITI), a collaboration between the pharmaceutical company Pfizer and the Edna McConnell Clark Foundation. A single dose of azithromycin—manufactured by Pfizer as Zithromax—could successfully treat active trachoma, a welcome change from the topical tetracycline ointment previously used, which required a six-week course, stung, and caused blurred vision. Azithromycin interferes with the *C. trachomatis* bacterium's ability to synthesize essential proteins, without which it cannot grow and replicate. For a disease that is recorded in Chinese documents dating from 2600 BCE and that is likely to be much older, azithromycin was the game changer. The drug's safety, stability, and effectiveness—together with Pfizer's commitment to donate the drug—had enabled the World Health Assembly in 1998 to adopt a resolution targeting the worldwide elimination of trachoma as a public health problem.

Solomon was sent to the northern region of Ghana "with a backpack full of money," he recalled, "about $5,000 in Ghanaian cedis to pay per diems to people and other expenses, which went across the White Volta River on top of a stack of six bikes in the bow of a dugout canoe, with a guy in the back paddling it with his flip-flops." Working in collaboration with Ghanaian ophthalmologist Dr. Maria Hagan and ophthalmic nurses Joe Akudibillah and Peter Abugri, Solomon taught volunteers to diagnose trachoma and treat it with Zithromax. The project's tremendous results inspired the Ghana Health Service to scale up the program to nationwide coverage. In 2009, Ghana was able to stop the mass drug administration (MDA) of Zithromax, and in 2018 the country completed WHO's multiyear process of validation that it had eliminated trachoma as a public health problem.

ITI's work changed too, expanding from five countries to forty. In 1999, ITI treated 100,000 people with Zithromax. In 2017, more than 87 million people received the antibiotic, and more than 222,000 underwent TT surgery. "Once you start supplying 120 million doses against a global need of 200 million, the number who need to be treated is going to come down progressively, and it won't be too long before those numbers meet," said Dr. Solomon. "We're not a million miles away from doing the whole job."

■　■　■

Besides treatment with azithromycin, cleanliness significantly helps break trachoma's transmission cycle: keeping one's face clean, using a latrine, and covering food and keeping it off the floor. But changing people's behavior is a more difficult task than explaining the benefits of taking a particular pill. Sanitation and hygiene practices differ according to local culture and the availability of necessary resources, including clean water. Farmers who are out in the field all day may see nothing wrong with defecating there—plus a loss of time and money walking to and from a latrine. Among the Maasai, a seminomadic people living in southern Kenya and northern Tanzania, it is taboo for women and children to see men defecating or even entering a latrine, and some latrines donated by NGOs have ended up as storage sheds.

If hygiene and sanitation can be improved, however, the benefits are manifold. After latrines became commonplace in the American South in the early 1900s, not only did hookworm disease subside, but so did giardiasis, hepatitis, typhoid fever, and other waterborne diseases. Washing one's face with water can make a huge difference. But, as Oliver Sokana, NTD program manager for the Solomon Islands, told me, "People believe if they barely have enough clean water to cook or drink, it would be a waste to use it washing your child's face." Dirty faces are sometimes perceived as a natural part of being young, not as a breeding ground for disease.

Helen Bokea, an NTD program specialist whose experience extends across Africa, described working in the Karamoja region in Uganda:

> One thing that struck me is that the women are relatively dirty compared to the men, who look very nicely turned out. I asked someone, "What's going on here?" The Karamojong men don't like their women being clean because they become attractive to other men. Their women will go for as long as a month without taking a bath. This is further complicated by lack of accessible water. The men don't like the women to go out of the home. The

men will take the animals to drink, so they get a chance to bathe. If you are trying to convince this woman that she needs to clean up, what are your chances of succeeding?

"There are a lot of cases still waiting," said Melese Kitu, a trachoma surgeon in Ethiopia, which in 2014 launched a fast-track initiative to clear the backlog of TT surgeries. "They are afraid of the surgery. There are other challenges, like the long distances to get to the health center. A challenge on our side is lack of transportation. We walk long distances in rural areas to give service." Nevertheless, Kitu said, "Doing this job has always been my dream. Even a single hair hurting their eyes and they feel a strong pain, a very bad pain. When I take that away, the relief I see in them makes me feel good. They are an old people, but they give you respect and blessings. I feel proud because of that. It's so good to see their happiness." He recalled one patient who "didn't expect she'd be cured. The pain was so bad for her that she didn't think her eyelash could be removed and that she would have a normal life. She never imagined she would be okay." At the postsurgery checkup, "she brought me honey and maize as a gift. She put it behind my chair. I saw it in the morning. It's a way to say, 'thanks for what you did.'"

Outside the West Gojjam health center where Kitu worked, an elderly man named Achenef Demilew awaited TT surgery. Through a translator, he said:

> During our fathers' time, it was very hard to get a solution, but now we have professionals so the problem is solved. Now, because of everybody's effort, we are getting better. Trachoma, it brings a very high pain around my eye and it makes me uncomfortable. The government has given us a medicine, but it only gives short-term relief. It makes me feel a lot of pain on the inside, then it makes me cry, and it makes my eyes too red.
>
> I got a message from around the village, so I came here to check

my eyes by the doctors. I was worried and felt stressed, because I thought the surgery may bring a bad outcome. I thought, it may bring good or bad? It may bring a darkness or brightness for me.

I came here because the government organized a community worker in my village. There are organizers around the community from women's affairs and local leadership. They travel around the community, and they told us to go to check our eyes. The organizers strongly advised us: "Don't lose this opportunity."

As long as the doctors came from the government, I believe I will get the surgery. I don't feel any fear. I feel so happy. Because of this, I'm really happy. I'll get my eye back. There are a lot of people around our village who are infected by trachoma. I came here by car, along with a lot of people from our village, around twenty-seven people. This number is from one single village. All together we are near seventy people. It will bring a full recovery for us.

In 1991, Morocco committed to eliminate trachoma by 2005. The country had been fighting the disease for nearly a hundred years, and prevalence had fallen as urban areas grew, the standard of living improved, and sanitation modernized. However, the disease still affected 5 percent of the country's population, mainly in the poorest rural provinces, as a 1992 survey revealed. In 1997, Morocco became the first country to implement on a national level WHO's four-pronged trachoma strategy, known as SAFE: surgery, antibiotics, facial cleanliness, and environmental improvement. A collaborative partnership was established among several ministries in the government (including health, education, water, and employment), international organizations, and local NGOs. A public education campaign was rolled out at mosques, schools, and community centers to encourage clean homes and personal hygiene. Outreach methods included videos, plays, meetings, pictures, posters, pamphlets, newspaper articles, and radio and television spots. A lesson on trachoma was incorporated into the primary-school curriculum. The government built latrines, drilled wells, and underwrote the cost of tens of thousands of TT surgeries, which were performed by mobile teams traveling to villages because people had limited means of transportation. Pfizer donated Zithromax worth more than $72 million. In 2006, Morocco was able to stop treatment, and it applied for validation that it had eliminated trachoma as a public health problem. (Elimination in this case means that the prevalence of active trachoma in children from 1 to 9 years old is less than 5 percent, and the prevalence of TT is less than 0.2 percent.)

Cambodia, Lao PDR, Mexico, Morocco, and Oman have all shown that with commitment and resources, trachoma can be eliminated as a public health problem. But this goal is more complicated in countries that are larger, less developed, or war-torn or whose governments lack money, staff, or technical resources. Sometimes a national NTD "department" is one overworked person who fills the roles of doctor, professor, and head of a prevention program. Simply finding the people who have trachoma can be a challenge. Community health workers are trained to go door to door to find trachoma cases, but, as Bokea said, "The patients will not just come out and say, 'I have TT.' Often you are looking for people you are not even sure exist."

"Mapping" is the process of locating a disease. It is used not only for streamlining treatment and prevention efforts, but as a baseline for measuring whether that work is effective. In the case of trachoma, mapping helps answer key questions. Is the disease a public health problem, or is it popping up sporadically? Is the level of infection high and only in targeted areas, or low and broad-based? Are there areas where treatment can be stopped because infection rates are sufficiently low after many years of treatment? What is the backlog of patients still needing surgery? Mapping is done by sending teams on the ground to systematically look for cases and report them to a central database. A certain number of villages per district and households per village are sampled to provide a statistically accurate representation of the disease at large.

According to the 2011 International Coalition for Trachoma Control report, "The End in Sight: 2020 INSight," from the 1990s until 2010, trachoma was mapped in 1,115 districts worldwide. At the end of that period, however, there were still 1,238 districts that were suspected of being endemic, but there were no reliable data on the disease's prevalence. Since this discrepancy existed, there was a good chance that even more infected districts remained unmapped.

The Global Trachoma Mapping Project (GTMP) was an international initiative funded by the UK's Department for International Development (DFID) for £10.6 million, with additional funds later contributed by USAID. The audacious plan—to complete a global baseline trachoma map in three years—was hatched by Danny Haddad, P. J. Hooper, Caroline Harper, and Anthony Solomon, who served as chief scientist for the project, while Tom Millar at Sightsavers was its operations director. "We anticipated that it would be 1,238 districts that needed mapping in thirty-four countries," Solomon recalled. "But once we started having very detailed conversations with Ministries of Health, more suspected endemic districts came out. More endemic countries than had been anticipated came out. Some of the countries that we thought needed mapping turned out not to need mapping. We ended up engaging with forty-nine countries, actively mapping in twenty-nine, and we mapped 1,546 districts in three years and three and a half weeks."

How did the team cover so much ground so quickly? The project's planners brought an inventive mind-set to the challenge and took into account and avoided common mapping pitfalls. The standardization of approaches, cooperation among multiple agencies, and health ministry ownership of the work and the resulting data were also extremely important. Finally, they utilized a tool that their trachoma-fighting predecessors could only dream of: the smartphone.

Each of the 611 field teams consisted of a grader and a recorder, both selected by the Ministry of Health and trained by the GTMP. To save time, the method of cascade training was deployed, whereby those who were trained could train others, in the field, using the eyes of real people rather than pictures. Moreover, the analysis was standardized internationally. "Before the GTMP, graders were not necessarily well trained," said Solomon. "That's not meant to be a pejorative comment. If you work somewhere where there isn't much active trachoma around, it's quite hard to arrange for people to know what active trachoma looks like. One of the big things done by GTMP was taking ophthalmologists from Yemen and Egypt and other low-prevalence environments to high-prevalence environments so that they saw what trachoma actually looks like."

Using a repurposed app originally built for lymphatic filariasis surveys, the recorder would take the household's GPS reading and enter the data collected by the grader. Using a flashlight and low-level magnification, the grader would examine each eye from the front and the side; a few blinks would reveal if the eyelashes were touching the cornea (indicating TT). Inverting the eyelid, the grader would look for signs of active trachoma: five or more white dots in the central part of the conjunctiva (trachomatous inflammation—follicular) or a "red and beefy" conjunctiva whose blood vessels weren't visible (trachomatous inflammation—intense). Each person could be examined in less than thirty seconds, including cleaning the grader's hands with alcohol-based hand gel. "Much of the time that is taken in doing a trachoma survey is walking house to house," Solomon said. The teams visited twenty to thirty villages per district and sampled approximately thirty households per village, meaning 2,000 to 4,000 people per district, for a total of 2.6 million people (or 5.2 million eyes).

As soon as the smartphone connected to a wireless or 3G network, its data zipped over to a secure server in the cloud. A full-time data manager based in Atlanta, Georgia, cleaned (i.e., found, corrected, and/or removed incorrect or incomplete pieces) and then submitted the data to the country's Ministry of Health for approval. The independent data manager was the only person who could change any data because, as Solomon explained, "it is impossible for program staff not to have a vested interest, and we did not want there to be questions about consistency or objectivity." The job of data management was therefore centralized to individuals without links to the programs themselves, while the data remained the property of the countries.

Ministries of Health are frequently reluctant to participate in disease surveys that require data to be public, because the results might make them look bad. But "when you point out that there are donors looking for opportunities to make a difference, and that by putting out there that you have this big problem and that treatment is not getting to the people, that represents an advertisement for additional support," Solomon said. "Governments are very willing to accept that. They understand that they can't actually do everything with current resources."

After the data were cleaned and approved, district-level prevalence categories were uploaded to the Trachoma Atlas, a public-interface website, "so that we could be sure that the public health decision that came from the mapping was accessible to people. It didn't disappear into an individual academic's computer or to a Ministry of Health person's computer and then you have that person move to another job and have the data be lost," Solomon said. "Most of this is funded through public money, particularly UK and US public money. It would be a tragedy if it were not available for public health application."

Mapping "has allowed the communities to understand what the background is," said Helen Bokea, who worked as the regional trachoma program coordinator for the international NGO called CBM. (Founded in 1908 as Christoffel-Blindenmission and known in English as Christian Blind Mission, the organization became CBM in 2007.) Bokea saw the power of mapping in Meru, Kenya: "The whole community, including the leadership, administration, and even some health-care workers, said, 'There is no trachoma in this community.' But because of a survey performed in 2004 by the Ophthalmic Services Unit of Kenya's Ministry of Health, we knew that there was trachoma there. Then you begin to find the people. You can imagine that without that mapping, and a community that is resisting that this disease even exists, it would have been really difficult, because then what would . . . enable you to keep pushing and saying, yes, there is work to be done."

When I asked Bokea if there was one person in her work who had especially touched her, she told me about Joyce, whom she'd met in western Uganda, where CBM was organizing outreach work and performing TT surgeries:

> She is a 50-year-old lady. She walks on all fours. This is the twenty-first century, yet there are communities where they are such poor people that they still have those challenges. She must have had polio when she was a child. Moving from point A to point B is not easy for such a person, but she had come to the outreach. Her daughter had brought her. She was a really beautiful woman. Despite all the challenges of life, she still looked good.

She was suffering from bilateral TT. Both her eyes needed surgery. She had heard about the outreach on the radio. Plus, their village health member had told her about it. The first time, two weeks earlier, there had been an outreach for cataract surgery. She came and was told, "Not today. The TT one is coming soon, so come back." She was determined to have that surgery.

She went in, had her surgery, and we took her home using the project vehicle. We said, "Let's see her home, and see what kind of wheelchair can we give her." It was quite far, a really bumpy road. I was thinking, "This lady sat on a motorbike all the way from that place to here." It was just that determination of hers to prevent herself from acquiring a second disability.

She lives in poverty. The windows of her house were covered permanently with iron sheets. That's partly because of the TT. The light affects people who are suffering from TT, so they tend to block windows completely. She is a mother of six children. A son of hers was there and her youngest child, plus there were grandchildren. They were dirty. Some had malnutrition. They had nasal and ocular discharge. She introduced us to her son who was 23 years old and dropped out of school because there was no money, and he is already the father of three children. You can see that the cycle of poverty goes on. Her husband doesn't support her much. She said he spends a lot of time drinking.

If you look at that environment and how dirty it is, and the fact that we had done the surgery and we are not doing antibiotics because they don't meet the threshold—but we haven't addressed the environment and the facial cleanliness. These small children, if they had trachoma, they could probably get it again. We are not cutting the transmission cycle.

We still leave them in that abject poverty. What are the chances they are going to have a better life? Hopefully, other sectors will come in, so that we are addressing the social determinants for health and not just focusing on treatment and leaving without considering how it will be sustained. Eventually you don't achieve what you intended to achieve. Hopefully, we can have a more holistic approach of eliminating NTDs.

Joyce perfectly, tragically demonstrates the tangle of NTDs and poverty. Sadly, this is not a new story. At the beginning of the twentieth century, more than 36,000 immigrants were denied entry to the United States after eye exams conducted on Ellis Island showed signs of trachoma. In San Francisco, immigrants from China, India, and Japan faced the same fate. During examinations, officers of the Public Health Service turned eyelids inside out using buttonhooks or their hands, both of which were often filthy. Various remedies were used to hide signs of the disease, from applying adrenaline to the eyeball to rubbing one's eyes with sugar cubes for six weeks. At the time, trachoma was endemic in overcrowded US and European cities, and officials wanted to limit the number of immigrants who would be unable to work or take care of themselves. Although less than 1 percent of immigrants were diagnosed with trachoma, the disease became a "trope of exclusion," as Ji-Hye Shin has written, providing a focal point for xenophobic fears that painted immigrants as dirty and more vulnerable to certain diseases. In 1891, the US Congress passed legislation stating that "the following classes of aliens shall be excluded from admission into the United States [including] . . . persons suffering from a loathsome or dangerous contagious disease." The first disease to be designated "loathsome or contagious" was trachoma. Subsequent years saw trachoma used to justify segregating Japanese students from white students in San Francisco schools and to deny reentry to Chinese Americans who had contracted trachoma while outside the United States.

By the 1950s, trachoma had disappeared from industrialized countries, largely due to better living conditions and improved sanitation. (The notable exception was among Australia's Aboriginal communities, where trachoma still exists.) Yet the disease remained entrenched in parts of the developing world. Within those at-risk populations, women are the most vulnerable. When a mother becomes blind, the eldest daughter often drops out of school to take over the household responsibilities. The daughter's education stops; her future opportunities and earning potential plummet. Trachoma alone accounts for at least $2.9 billion in economic losses every year. Dr. Youssef Chami Khazraji, head of Morocco's National Blindness Control Program, described his government's position during an early phase of its trachoma campaign: "We now recognized that trachoma at the level of these regions is not strictly a medical problem; it is essentially the reflection of a socioeconomic problem. . . . In sum, the enemy to combat is not chlamydia but poverty."

■   ■   ■

In 2013, one year after observing Nieba's surgery, I met Susan, an elderly member of the Maasai, who are known for their beautiful, intricately beaded bracelets and necklaces. The market for the jewelry is robust, thanks in part to tourists on safari in Kenya's Maasailand. Susan's beadwork was masterly, and the income it had generated had supported her family for years.

Susan had undergone TT surgery, though not without considerable doubts. People resist for many reasons—superstition, acceptance of their blindness, misunderstanding, fear. Helen Bokea told me of a Ugandan woman who thought her sight would be restored, and when it wasn't—because she had cataracts, which had already affected her vision—the woman railed against the procedure to her community. Some women stay away because they don't have a nice enough dress to wear to the surgery, Bokea said. Blind, Susan would lose her income. She would change from supporting her family to being dependent on them. Her family would suffer too, because there would be less money. She decided to have the surgery.

Thrilled with the results, Susan became an outspoken advocate, going from village to village to testify to the benefits of the surgery. Community health workers traveling with Susan wore large colorful wraps on which were illustrations of two homesteads. One was a breeding ground for trachoma. The ideal homestead showed dishes kept off the ground, a latrine in use, children without flies in their eyes, and a leaky tin (aka tippy tap), a water jug suspended from a tree. A basic form of plumbing, the jug has a stick plugging a small hole in it. Removing the stick lets water drip slowly, just enough to use with soap for face and hand washing. This simple device helps prevent a disease that wrecks lives.

Midway through my conversation with Susan, she took a call on her cell phone: an order for beadwork. She was the embodiment of old and new: a tall, elegant woman dressed in the brilliant fabrics and scarves that are customary among the Maasai, standing outside her home made of mud and stone with dirt floors and a thatched roof, a successful businesswoman and entrepreneur on her cell phone closing a deal. Trachoma—which crippled Napoleon's army in Egypt in the early 1800s and spread around the world during the Crusades and the Peloponnesian War—had reached Susan. But she had undergone TT surgery. She would take azithromycin. She would keep herself and her children clean. This modern woman had beaten an ancient disease.

CHAPTER THREE

Big Consequences from Small Things

An impressive collection of microscopes was on display in Dr. William C. Campbell's living room in North Andover, Massachusetts. He has a sixth sense for finding the instruments, his wife, Mary, said, and he can spot them from outside a shop though they might be half hidden in a corner. The oldest dates to the late eighteenth century. Campbell pointed out his student microscope, which he took to Trinity College in Dublin. His training there laid the groundwork for his graduate studies at the University of Wisconsin-Madison, where his central project—on liver fluke in sheep and cattle—started a career in parasites. He was drawn to their "grottiness," as he put it, as well as the extraordinary complexity of their life cycles.

His Nobel Prize was tucked away in his office, where I spotted a cardboard box unceremoniously labeled "Stuff from Stockholm," which was filled with newspaper clippings and memorabilia—tickets, schedules, menus, programs—from the Nobel week. Awarded in 2015, the prize honored Campbell and Dr. Satoshi Ōmura for their contributions to the treatment of diseases caused by roundworms; the most high-profile component of their work was the use of ivermectin for control of onchocerciasis (river blindness). Since 1987, the drug has been donated by Merck Sharp & Dohme (MSD, which operates as Merck & Co. in the United States and Canada), first to treat river blindness and later to prevent lymphatic filariasis (LF). Every year, 250 million people receive ivermectin. Since donations began, more than 2 billion treatments have been distributed.

"In the context of river blindness, I had a very small role," Campbell said. "It happened to be that there are big consequences to some small things."

■   ■   ■

"A tiny fly breeds in the river of northern Ghana," the late Sir John Wilson wrote in his 1963 book, *Travelling Blind*. "People who see it skimming over the water say that it is a beautiful thing with its black and silver colouring. It is called *Simulium damnosum* and it causes blindness on an unbelievable scale."

With a bite into human flesh, the *Simulium damnosum*, or black fly, can deliver via its saliva parasitic worms. These worms mature inside nodules under the skin; some grow to twenty inches or longer. Then they mate, with females producing 500 to 1,500 off-spring daily. In endemic areas (which include West, Central, and East Africa, parts of Latin America, and Yemen), a person may host up to 100 million worm larvae (called microfilariae), which cause intense, relentless itching. Eventually another black fly bites, picks up some microfilariae, and during a subsequent bite transfers them to another host, where the worms repeat the cycle.

Some of the worms wiggle and wander in the skin. Some wind up in the host's eye. When the microfilariae die there, they cause an inflammatory response in the host, which creates opacities over the cornea. Over time, multiple opacities form and merge, blocking out light. In endemic regions, some people start losing their sight in their 20s and are blind by 40.

Another outcome is onchocerca skin disease (aka craw-craw), in which the inflammation from the dying microfilariae causes pigmentary changes, thickening, and eventual loss of elasticity of the skin. The nodules that house the adult worms can be felt under the skin and are sometimes visible.

In 1947, the British Crown sent John Wilson on a ten-month tour of West Africa to investigate blindness and disabilities in its colonies. Blind himself as the result of a childhood accident in chemistry class, Wilson was appalled at what he encountered. As his widow, Lady Jean Wilson, told me, "To him, his blindness was a confounded nuisance and nothing more, but [in Africa], children were hidden away, disgraced, and blind people were considered incapable of anything at all." In a report on a 1950 trip to Ghana, included in *Travelling Blind*, Wilson wrote:

> At Nakong, fifty people met us on the muddy bank of the swollen river. They were like specimens from a medical museum and behind them their village lay as silent as a cemetery. The clinical records showed that a tenth of the people in this village and a sixth of the adult males were totally blind.
>
> They answered our questions quietly but asked none themselves. Yes, there was much blindness; every family had blind people. No, there was no cure for blindness; it came from the river when foam was on the water. Of course there were many black flies; anyone could hear them humming through the compounds in the evening and if you killed one there were a thousand more.
>
> They showed us their houses with tiny entrances, probably protection against animals. They had not bothered to clear the rotting vegetation from the paths and, as they shuffled slowly behind us, it was difficult to believe that they had enough energy left to do so. We stood aside to allow two blind men to pass. They were walking one behind the other, both holding a long piece of bamboo at the front end of which a child was leading the way.
>
> Along the bank it is said that you can find ruins of fifteen deserted villages buried under the high grass. At one large ruin the

interpreter remembered the names of eight people who had lived there; two young ones emigrated in their canoes and the others died from some cause or other until only two were left, a blind man and an old woman. They had disappeared after the bad harvest two years previously.

We went on to Vare, a few miles from Nakong. The tax register showed that it had thirty-two inhabitants; there had been 174 at the 1931 census. Outside that village, at the point where the track ended, a piece of rope joined two trees. We were told that it was to guide women to the water-hole.

At another place a young man, sitting cross-legged beside the river, was mending a fish-trap. We had been told that he was blind, but it was not until he ignored our greeting that we realized he was also deaf.

As we left those villages I felt sick and angry and was possessed with the urgent need to get something done about this situation. That little had been done in the past was due not to apathy but to uncertainty about the facts and to the physical difficulties of the task.

In response to what he had witnessed, Wilson formed the British Empire Society for the Blind, which financed and produced the first standardized survey of the causes and distribution of blindness in West Africa. The results were published in two books: *Blindness in West Africa* by ophthalmologist Dr. F. C. Rodger and *Simulium and Onchocerciasis in the Northern Territories of the Gold Coast* by entomologist Dr. Geoffrey Crisp. Some of the blindness resulted from trachoma or cataracts, but most was caused by onchocerciasis. The locals "thought it had something to do with the river, but they didn't know," said Lady Jean. Entire villages with good, arable land were being abandoned. Families faced an awful choice: stay and go blind, or save their sight but give up their means of growing food and earning money. She recalled her first visit to an onchocerciasis-endemic region in 1952: "We went through the cocoa plantations, through the busy hubbub of African villages, and then we came to this awful silence. Deserted villages, a few scraggly crops, a little huddle of round, thatched mud houses. These people were so debilitated. Not just blind or going blind, but they've got these awful lumps all over them. The only things that were active were the insects on the floor." Deficiencies in vitamin A and parasites of the gastrointestinal tract were undoubtedly contributing to the widespread lethargy.

During this trip through the "country of the blind," the Wilsons' car broke down near a riverbed. "The driver went for help," said Lady Jean. "We sat half a day in this broiling heat with the windows up. All the flies were pinging up from the river." As they discussed the empty villages, the overwhelming blindness, and the role of onchocerciasis, Lady Jean said, "I can't say it. I can't spell it. How can I raise funds for it?" Looking outside, she said, "Could we call it river blindness?"

Speaking to me sixty-three years later, she elaborated, "If you knew nothing about it, and we said, 'Will you give to onchocerciasis?' what would you know? To give, you've got to understand it first, haven't you?"

The British Empire Society for the Blind—which changed its name to the Royal Commonwealth Society for the Blind and is now known publicly as Sightsavers—worked to help visually impaired people around the world live independently and to eliminate preventable blindness (which accounts for 80 percent of all blindness worldwide). The society established schools and training centers to break down stigmas and get people with blindness back to work. "The blind men were brought from their villages and trained how to do crops, and then we escorted them back and got them set up on their land again," said Lady Jean, who was the society's photographer and main fundraiser. "They were usually better farmers than the other people." Mobile surgical units could often restore vision loss caused by cataracts, but river blindness, whose pathology had been pieced together in the late nineteenth and early twentieth centuries, remained intractable. Prevention and treatment did not exist.

■ ■ ■

In March 1974, a shipment of fifty-four isolated microbes arrived at MSD in Rahway, New Jersey. The microbes—bacteria—had been scooped up by Satoshi Ōmura from under a tree bordering a golf course in his home neighborhood in Ito, Japan. Ōmura always carried a plastic bag in his pocket so that he could take soil samples from places that looked promising for bacteria. Why soil near a golf course? "There are certain places," Bill Campbell told me, "for example, under shady trees near open spaces, where microbiologists get a feel for a good sample. It's like fishermen: I think if we go further upstream . . ."

At the Kitasato Institute, Ōmura and his colleagues isolated and grew colonies of the different bacteria extracted from the soil. Some of the bacteria were recognizable and therefore irrelevant. Kitasato and MSD (with which Kitasato shared isolates with "unusual morphological characteristics") were looking for unknown microbes. The discovery in the early twentieth century of the first antibiotic, penicillin—a chemical compound made by a fungus—had been the starter gun on a decades-long race to find other microbes with antibacterial products that could be used to treat human infections. The miracle of antibiotics is that they selectively harm the infecting agent while leaving the patient relatively unscathed. With antibiotics, infections and diseases that had been death sentences—pneumonia, tuberculosis, meningitis, strep throat—suddenly were not. By the late 1960s, however, the search for new antibiotics had slowed almost to a halt, with medical leaders erroneously claiming that infectious disease had been conquered. Still, MSD had agreements to receive microbial isolates from institutes around the world. Beyond antibiotics for human use, the company was looking for ways to fight growth-inhibiting infections and parasites in livestock.

A year after Kitasato isolate number OS3153 became MSD isolate MA-4680, it and Ōmura's fifty-three other microbes were up for an assay, which is a test to see what effect, if any, they might have against anything. The MSD parasitologists tested one isolate after another: they would grow a bacterium in a broth, freeze-dry the fermented broth, and add it to the feed of a mouse infected with a particular parasite. Whether the specific bacterium had produced anything "active"—anything that killed—was determined by the presence or absence of worms in the mouse's intestine and worm eggs in its feces. "Part of drug discovery involves a lot of routine screening and testing," said Campbell. "I found that routine work not only very satisfying, but also it presented opportunities to do some fun side stuff."

The "fun side stuff" included experiments in trichinellosis ("I spent an awful lot of time working on that disease, which was of no interest to the company whatsoever"). Campbell recalled "an excitement" and a "friendly competitiveness" between MSD and other companies. "For the entire workday, you're just doing research, and it's absolutely terrific." When Campbell succeeded Ashton Cuckler as head of parasitology, his budget, about $1 million, was one of the biggest at MSD. Still, "failure was the default position." The team had tested 40,000 microbial isolates prior to MA-4680.

Since the scientists didn't know what the microbes might be producing—perhaps something, perhaps nothing—they had no way to know how much to give the mice. "A goop," Campbell said.

The control mouse got none. "Other mice got other goops. . . . We fed to them an unknown amount of an unknown substance that might not be there." He added, "The thing about this assay is that it could have been operated fifty years earlier, had it been thought of. The concept, in fact, was original. Technically it could have been done, except that it had not been devised. Scientifically it could have been devised, but it wasn't. There was a mental block—a methodological block—but it wasn't a technical, scientific one. Nobody had thought there was a way around that impasse. This was fresh thinking on the part of the Merck staff. There was no breakthrough cutting-edge science. It was all such simple stuff."

The mouse that for six days was fed MA-4680 nearly died before the end of the assay. It hadn't eaten much and had lost weight, but it was free of worms. A battery of examinations and tests by other departments—microbiology, biochemistry, toxicology, pharmacology—revealed the identity and mechanism of the anthelmintic (anti-worm) activity. A chemical compound was acting as a nerve poison against the worms. A new species of Streptomyces bacterium was producing the poison, and the poison, designated C-076, was a new chemical and biological class of antiparasitic agent. "It has a degree of potency quite unheard-of against parasitic worms," Campbell explained. "It has a breadth of spectrum quite unprecedented, especially [since] it includes a number of arthropods and a huge range of roundworms." Even at a concentration of 0.0003 percent, C-076 could rid a mouse of worms.

"A new name was needed," Bill Campbell wrote in "The Genesis of the Antiparasitic Drug Ivermectin." "I proposed *avermecticin*, the ending '-icin' indicating, by convention, an actinomycete origin, and the rest of the word suggesting antagonism toward worms (vermes) and ectoparasites. Dr. Jerry Birnbaum proposed that the name be trimmed to *avermectin*."

Avermectin refers to a group of eight similar chemical structures, each with its own compositional characteristics and varying efficacy against different worms. MSD's chemists manipulated one of these structures, avermectin B1a, so it would work against the largest number of worms. Because the chemists had added hydrogen, the first name proposed for the new creation was hyvermectin. Eventually, it was called ivermectin.

Over the next few years, the drug was tested in dogs, sheep, cattle, rabbits, ferrets, and jirds. In minute amounts, it proved active against an enormous range of parasitic worms found throughout the gastrointestinal tract, including worms that had proven resistant to earlier anthelmintics. It also worked against worms found outside the intestinal tract as well as free-living insect pests and parasitic insects, including flour beetles, ear mites, mange mites, and sucking lice. Fortunately, ivermectin was not active against the adult stage of dog heartworm—killing these worms often also kills the dog—but it did work against the worms' preadult stage with extreme efficacy and no side effects. If you have ever given a dog a heartworm pill, you have likely handled ivermectin.

It was, the scientists at MSD realized, the most potent anthelmintic ever known. It could be given at very low doses. It could be administered in a variety of ways, including orally, by subcutaneous shot, and by external application. The drug had a long shelf life and didn't require special handling, for example, refrigeration. Most important, the host species tolerated the drug, a good indicator of its safety. In 1981 MSD put ivermectin on the market under the trade name Ivomec. By 1984 it was the number one animal pharmaceutical in the world.

■　■　■

In 1978, Lyndia Slayton Blair, a junior parasitologist, senior technician, and assistant to Bill Campbell and Dr. John Eggerton, had the idea to test ivermectin on worms in horses. Having read a recently published paper that stated the high prevalence of onchocerca larvae in horses, Blair suggested adding a skin snip test to the necropsy protocol during an assay run by Eggerton. The result: ivermectin was active against the microfilariae of *Onchocerca cervicalis* in horses. After receiving Eggerton's report, Campbell asked Dr. Bruce Copeman, a veterinary parasitologist in Australia, to try ivermectin against *Onchocerca gutturosa* in cattle. Again, the drug killed the larval worms.

For twenty-five years, Campbell had taught a class on human parasitology at New York Medical College, which had added to his awareness of developments (or lack thereof) in human parasitic diseases. With evidence that ivermectin was active against two species of onchocerca, he sent a memorandum to his boss, Jerry Birnbaum, proposing that ivermectin be tested in humans to see if it would work against onchocerciasis.

At the time, the only large-scale response to river blindness was vector control: killing the black flies that carry the *Onchocerca volvulus* worm from human to human. The Onchocerciasis Control Program (OCP) had launched in 1974—the same year the fifty-four microbial isolates were sent from Japan to New Jersey. Through aerial spraying of insecticide on fly breeding sites throughout West Africa's Volta River basin, the program aimed to reduce the blinding form of the disease carried by the savanna black flies. Since aerial spraying would be ineffective in dense vegetation, the forest black fly, whose disease causes more itching than blindness, was not targeted. When OCP began, in some savanna areas more than 60 percent of the population was infected with the parasite, and more than half of men over 40 years old had lost their sight.

The program had been launched by World Bank president (and former US secretary of defense) Robert McNamara. Led by scientists from France, the UK, the US, and the endemic countries, OCP was a joint effort of the World Bank, WHO, the UN Development Programme, the Food and Agriculture Organization, and donor countries Canada, France, Federal Republic of Germany, the Netherlands, the UK, the US, and others. Designed to last twenty years, after which it would be run by local governments, the program sent teams into the field to find fly breeding sites. Based on their data, which were communicated weekly via radio to headquarters in Burkina Faso, pilots in eleven helicopters and two fixed-wing aircraft sprayed the larvicide temephos into the water.

Professor Daniel Boakye (bo-AH-chee), one of the world's foremost black fly experts, joined OCP in 1984 as part of the field team that looked for sites and also collected and studied the flies. "Going into the breeding site is a bit scary; some of the water is up to your neck," said Boakye. Female flies deposit eggs on rocks, branches, and foliage just below the surface of fast-flowing rivers, whose movement provides the aquatic stages with oxygen. Two to three days later, larvae hatch from the eggs; they remain in place for eight to ten days, growing by filtering nutrients from the water. During this window of vulnerability, insecticide sprayed into the river upstream of the site passes through the larvae's filter and into their gut, killing them.

"You can get larvae breeding on supports on the edges of the stream or sometimes in the middle, where you have rocks and other things that break the water. You have to check all these areas." Boakye grew up in Ghana and attended the Kwame Nkrumah University of Science and Technology before earning a master's degree in medical entomology and applied parasitology at the University of Jos in Nigeria. He joined OCP as an intern and later became its cytotaxonomist, in charge of identifying black fly species (there are twelve in West Africa alone).

"Sometimes you have to cross the river. It's very high. It's very fast. If you try to do it without a rope, you'll get swept away,"

Boakye said. A few people drowned during these efforts, and there were some helicopter and aircraft crashes, one of which killed everyone on board. But "you never really thought about the risks," which were mitigated by a strong sense of pride that they were doing something to alleviate the widespread blindness. "One of the emotional things is seeing a positive breeding site," he said, "because then you have identified the source of the problem." He described OCP as "one of the best programs I've worked with," adding, "there was a sense of family."

Aquatic and fish biologists rigorously monitored the impact of temephos and other insecticides on "nontarget organisms" to minimize environmental damage. Local villagers, however, wanted a demonstrative explanation. "You say you're going to put insecticide in the rivers and you get apprehension, especially if they are fisher folk," Boakye said. "So when you collect adult flies and you get an infected fly, you ask the village leader to come and have a look at it. You would be outdoors, everyone crowded around. They've never looked into a microscope before. You see a live worm moving around. Then they say, 'Wow, this is really something.'" Sometimes the team would put under the microscope a skin snip, a one- or two-milligram piece of someone's skin. "You see hundreds of parasites," he said. First, people would gasp. Then, "you would get that sort of facial expression: so, if this small piece of skin is teeming with this number of parasites, imagine what it means that your whole body is covered with this." Finally, "everybody wanted a skin snip." Once they understood what was happening, the communities were appreciative because aside from reducing blindness, OCP had decreased, if not annihilated, the flies, whose bites are very painful. When I asked if he'd ever been bitten, Boakye laughed. "That was part of the job! You got bitten many times."

In the 1980s, OCP doubled its operational area to 1.2 million square kilometers of land and 30,000 miles of river, and added four countries to the original seven (in all: Benin, Burkina Faso, Côte d'Ivoire, Ghana, Guinea, Guinea-Bissau, Mali, Niger, Senegal, Sierra Leone, Togo). The expansion, which was needed to counter the reinvasion of black flies, led to a tremendous cost increase. However, current donors stepped up and more donors were found. Another challenge was resistance to temephos. The problem was solved by rotating insecticides. The program's mandate had always been *control*, that is, lowering the prevalence to a manageable level. "Nobody at that time had the belief that you could eliminate the disease," Boakye said.

■　■　■

"I was a country doctor, and I was going to do what I thought was right," said Dr. Roy Vagelos, who, as head of MSD's research laboratories, read Bill Campbell's 1978 proposal to test ivermectin against river blindness and encouraged him to pursue a form that could be used in humans.

There were risks and obstacles. The only known medicine for river blindness at the time was diethylcarbamazine (DEC), which required an intense treatment schedule and occasionally caused severe, life-threatening reactions. Would ivermectin be different? Almost none of the people who needed ivermectin could pay for it. Their governments, too, had limited funds. Many were contending with war and starvation. "The marketing people said they would find a price that was affordable," said Vagelos.

In 1980, a coin toss gave Dr. Mohammed Aziz the assignment of overseeing the first human trials. A year later, thirty-two infected men were brought to the university hospital in Dakar, Senegal, and given various doses of ivermectin or placebos. Skin snips six weeks later showed clear results: patients who had been given fifty micrograms per kilogram of body weight of ivermectin showed either total elimination or near elimination of detectable microfilariae, with minor side effects.

Vagelos approved further trials, but MSD needed a partner. Who was going to buy the drug for endemic countries? Who would distribute it? Soon after sending his proposal to Birnbaum and Vagelos, Bill Campbell had approached WHO, inviting its assistance. The leadership at WHO declined, arguing that treatment for river blindness needed a drug that would kill the macrofilariae (the adult worm), not a microfilaricide like ivermectin. After the first phase of human trials, Vagelos, who had become MSD's chair and CEO, approached WHO with another invitation, which was also declined. In a letter to the *Lancet*, which had published Aziz's findings in the Senegal trials, WHO's André C. Rougemont wrote, "At this stage ivermectin, although representing a new class of microfilaricide, brings no really new or interesting feature to the treatment of onchocerciasis." The WHO leadership was, as Campbell put it, "a victim of their own expertise. They just could not accept that this thing that was acting against the microfilariae could be useful, especially when the only other one [DEC] was so disastrous."

Vagelos appealed to the US government. Deputy Secretary of State John Whitehead "was particularly excited." The estimated price for treating river blindness in Africa was about $2 million for the first year. "Walking out of his office, his aide said, 'Dr. Vagelos, that is such a wonderful story you tell. But you know something? It's not in the budget for this year.'"

Because there is no river blindness in the United States, the Food and Drug Administration would not test ivermectin—manufactured by MSD as Mectizan—so MSD filed the drug with French regulatory authorities, which were notoriously reluctant to bring new drugs to the market. "To my chagrin—because we did not have a plan for distribution—they called and said they were going to approve the drug," Vagelos said. "Like, they called on a Thursday and they were going to approve it on Monday."

On October 22, 1987, at a press conference in Washington, DC, Vagelos, flanked by Senators Bill Bradley, Frank Lautenberg, and Ted Kennedy, announced that MSD would give the drug to countries with endemic river blindness: "as much as needed, for as long as needed." "There was no way that we'd have that drug and not get it out to people," he said. In the rush of the approval and announcement, however, he didn't run his plan by MSD's board. It didn't cross his mind to do so, he told me years later. At the next board meeting, he asked if anyone would have made a different decision. The answer was a unanimous no. "I never did look to see what the cost of the program would be," Vagelos said. "Of course, I never envisioned how big it would be."

■   ■   ■

MSD was willing to manufacture and donate ivermectin—but how would the drug reach the people who needed it? OCP's mobile teams began delivering the drug in 1988, but the program's mandate was for eleven African countries, and river blindness was in nineteen. Ivermectin needed to reach hundreds of thousands of extremely remote villages. Moreover, because ivermectin kills *micro*filariae but not *macro*filariae, the drug needs to be taken annually beyond the life-span of the adult worms, which can be as long as fifteen years; only then is a person worm-free and no longer part of the parasite's transmission cycle.

The African Programme for Onchocerciasis Control (APOC) was established in 1995 to address this daunting challenge. APOC was built on the model of OCP and was initially based on distribution by nongovernmental development organizations (NGDOs), which were already distributing several million ivermectin treatments per year in the worst affected areas. These NGDOs contributed a significant amount toward APOC's implementation costs, as well as technical advice in the field.

Dr. Uche Amazigo, a public health specialist, had combined her teaching and lecturing at the University of Nigeria, Nsukka, with field visits to rural health clinics. "I would drive my private vehicle to villages and talk to women on health issues, on menstruation, on cleaning and hygiene," Amazigo told me.

> It was during one of those visits that I met Agnes, a young lady. She was pregnant, about 19 years old at that time. She had been sent away by her husband because she had lesions all over her body, unsightly lesions, itching lesions. The pregnancy exacerbated the lesions. Out of compassion, I requested her bills be sent to me and paid for her medication. I would go every Monday to see how far along she was. I didn't want her to lose her pregnancy, and she didn't. My master's student had taken a skin snip from Agnes and then examined it and found microfilarial worms. I did not know, the first time I saw Agnes, that she had river blindness. I didn't know what it was, because the lesions were just so bad and itching. At that time, in the '90s, the emphasis was on blinding onchocerciasis. Nobody was paying attention to the skin disease.

Agnes was a catalyst for research by Amazigo and others, which demonstrated the stigmatization of people with onchocerca skin disease. Women with the condition frequently do not marry, or are divorced by their husbands, or marry later in life. An enormous amount of labor is lost due to itching or erroneous fears of contagion. Amazigo recalled:

> To reach Agnes and to understand the social implications of river blindness on women in rural Nigeria, to understand their hidden stories, I had to register to become a member of Agnes's rural women's community and attend their meetings on weekends: sit

on the floor with them, eat what they were eating, and just be one of them. So when I came to APOC, I was convinced that bringing the people into the process and making them part of the solution would be the best way to distribute ivermectin. When APOC pushed for community self-treatment, later called community-directed treatment with ivermectin [CDTI], I had to champion it because I was entirely convinced that was the way forward.

Through a series of meetings, proposals, workshops, and field studies organized by OCP and the task force Onchocerciasis Operations Research (OOR), a group of African researchers found a way to distribute ivermectin that was simple, effective, and sustainable. "We had an open mind to this," Dr. Amazigo said, recalling an OOR meeting in Mali. "We decided: let us just ask one simple research question, and that question should be directed to the community. We asked the community to design a strategy themselves. We decided to compare the strategy designed by the communities with the strategy designed by the health system. These two strategies were attempted in different countries. And we realized that the strategy designed by the community had better coverage."

A 2007 publication by the African Programme for Onchocerciasis Control and WHO describes how a village would initiate CDTI:

The process begins with an informal enquiry: a health worker pays a visit to [a] community chief and arranges a meeting with the facilitation team and entire community. At this forum, the concept of community-directed treatment with ivermectin is explained. The community is then given time to select individuals they want to put forward for training as [community drug] distributors (CDDs), who are village members chosen according to the priorities of the community.

Once this decision is made, the community informs the health worker of a preferred date for training the new CDDs. Once this instruction is done—usually in a group with representatives from several different communities—the newly trained CDDs conduct a census of their community, record the results in a notebook and keep a copy in the home of the village or community leader.

The community as a whole decides on month[s] and dates of ivermectin distribution, which the CDD communicates to the health worker/facilitation team. If possible, the CDDs collect ivermectin tablets from the nearest health post on a date previously agreed with health workers. When the drugs are in the possession of the CDD, distribution can begin.

CDDs monitor adverse reactions and treat cases of minor reactions where possible. Any difficult or severe cases are referred to the nearest health facility. After the drug has been given out, the CDDs must complete the treatment record notebook or form and return a copy to the health post from which the ivermectin was collected. These records are monitored by health workers during any future visits to the village and the health post records are updated accordingly.

Amazigo recounts this history in "The Development of Community Directed Treatment for Tackling River Blindness," a chapter in *African Health Leaders*:

The CDTI strategy put communities at the heart of disease management in ways that no public health programme had done before. The premise was simple: it empowered the communities to take full responsibility for ivermectin delivery, by their own decisions as to how, when, and by whom the ivermectin treatment should be administered. The community directed distributors (CDDs) would go from household to household and from village to village delivering ivermectin on an unpaid voluntary basis. In the rural isolated populations or conflict-torn countries where health systems were always weak and under-resourced,

CDTI proved to be one of Africa's most successful programmes in reducing onchocercal disease at low cost.

"If I hadn't met Agnes, I don't know what would have happened," said Amazigo, who served as APOC's scientific lead (1996–2005) and then as its director (2005–2011). After ivermectin cleared her lesions, Agnes became a CDD herself. "Over time," Amazigo recalled, "with the donation of ivermectin that's now spread across Africa, and with APOC in place, people began to understand that those lesions are caused by this disease, and that taking ivermectin would clear them."

■ ■ ■

Between 1987 and 2017, more than 2.7 billion treatments were provided by the Mectizan Donation Program (MDP), the public-private partnership established by MSD with the Task Force for Global Health, and distributed by APOC, Ministries of Health, and the active NGDO community focused on supporting river blindness control efforts. In 1998, MDP expanded its mandate to include donating ivermectin to treat LF. Since the program's inception, MDP has supported national programs in twenty-nine countries in Africa, six countries in Latin America, and Yemen. Some donors have been fighting river blindness for decades. Kuwait, for example, was one of the first donors to OCP, continued to contribute support through APOC, and now provides support to APOC's successor, the Expanded Special Project for Elimination of NTDs (ESPEN).

Colombia, Ecuador, Guatemala, and Mexico have seen river blindness eliminated. As Daniel Boakye pointed out, however, there are "vastly different numbers in the African context compared to the Americas. In Colombia, the total population at risk was just 1,366. Nowhere in the African situation will you have such low numbers, even within a district." Other challenges include the possibility of the evolution of drug resistance in the parasite, achieving high coverage rates, and cross-border transmission.

The funding landscape continues to evolve, with important new donors joining the efforts. In 2017, Sheikh Mohammed bin Zayed bin Sultan Al-Nahyan, the crown prince of Abu Dhabi, established the Reaching the Last Mile Fund, a multidonor fund to be managed by the END Fund, which will raise and disburse $100 million over ten years, with the goal of eliminating river blindness in Chad, Ethiopia, Mali, Niger, Senegal, Sudan, and Yemen. According to Dr. Mona Hammami, a senior manager at the Office of Strategic Affairs for the Abu Dhabi Crown Prince Court, three of the countries selected for the fund are "close to the end": Mali, Niger, and Senegal. Two countries—Sudan and Yemen—are conflict zones. "We did know that there's a huge risk that in many of these conflict zones, we might not reach the end game, but at least starting it is extremely important," Hammami said. At the time of the fund's launch, $20 million had been pledged by the crown prince, and the Gates Foundation had committed up to $20 million, or 20 percent of the fund. Reaching the Last Mile, which will also target LF, is a milestone—for funding, but also for long-term dedication to proving that the elimination of river blindness is possible in Africa.

Merck Sharp & Dohme set a new standard. Today most major pharmaceutical companies not only donate drugs but commit R&D resources to finding the next generation of treatments. More than $4 billion of NTD medicines are donated per year by Eisai, Gilead, GlaxoSmithKline, Johnson & Johnson, Merck KGaA, MSD, Novartis, Pfizer, and Sanofi. With the price of drugs and other commodities playing a part in the cost of global health interventions, these contributions will make it possible in the coming years to control and eliminate intestinal worms, LF, river blindness, schistosomiasis, and other NTDs, such as leprosy, sleeping sickness, and visceral leishmaniasis. In 2016, more than a billion people received drugs to treat one or more of these diseases.

■ ■ ■

Ivermectin was a thread of possibility in a knot of obstacles. The answer to an otherwise unbeatable disease existed, though it might never have been found if Ōmura had not scooped up that soil. If the parasitology group had not been determined to continue the empirical approach—trial and error—despite pressure to adopt a more biochemical approach. If Blair had not suggested and Eggerton had not run the test for *Onchocerca cervicalis*. If Campbell had not taught human parasitology. If the CEO of MSD had not been a physician, attuned to human health beyond costs. If Amazigo had not met Agnes. Luck played a large role—though *not* serendipity, which, as Bill Campbell has pointed out, means finding something other than what you are looking for. "There is one element in this that is sheer serendipity, which is horse bots," he said. "We had not infected these horses with horse bot, we didn't know they had horse bot, but because we gave them ivermectin and then these dead horse bots were passed in the feces, then we had the diagnosis and the treatment all at once, neither of which we had any idea that we were going to find."

The luck of ivermectin has depended on an enormous amount of labor and preparation, marked by a few pivotal moments. In my conversations with Lady Jean Wilson, Bill Campbell, Daniel Boakye, Roy Vagelos, and Uche Amazigo, I was struck by their commitment to search for solutions, whether abstract (increased knowledge and awareness of river blindness) or tangible (finding black fly breeding sites). Often taking great personal and professional risks, they persevered, never knowing the outcome. "The great thing was to allow teamwork to happen," said Campbell, who, in his Nobel lecture and elsewhere, has emphasized that in accepting the prize, he was the representative of a "team of teams." "Everybody was wanting to make this succeed," he told me. When I heard him speak at MSD's headquarters in New Jersey, he put up a slide with the names of 125 people who were part of the effort.

"How do you describe what you did?" I asked. He broke his role into three parts. The first was as a scientist who was "big" on assay methodology: studying and manipulating parasites under lab conditions in order to devise and improve ways of detecting new active substances ("for example, by using one kind of parasite as a surrogate for another, or studying the best phase in the life cycle of the parasite to permit detection of activity"). The second was administrative: as the director of parasitology, "I didn't screw up what happened. There was a lot going on in my department and it all seemed to go okay." And the third—"the one that had big consequences"—"simply was calling attention to prospects in river blindness. That is why I went to see my boss and I told him about the disease and why the new drug candidate might work."

His last remark reminded me of Lady Jean's description of the society's early work, a description applicable to much of my own work decades later. It remains a cornerstone of ending NTDs: "We alerted people that there was such a need."

CHAPTER FOUR

Empowerment and Humility

Behind the health center in Merawi, a modest village in northwestern Ethiopia, about seventy-five men and women sat on benches in and around an open-air, tin-roofed shelter, which was stabilized by a pole connected to a tall tree on which were posted notices and announcements. The group came here about every six weeks, some traveling for hours, to have their feet washed, an act that was difficult, if not impossible, for them to accomplish themselves because of the massive enlargement of their legs. Lymphedema occurs when the vessels of the lymphatic system become dysfunctional, resulting in swollen limbs and genitalia. Some of the men and women around me had elephantiasis, an advanced form of lymphedema in which the skin is tough, lacks elasticity, and becomes so swollen it folds over itself. These conditions are symptoms of either podoconiosis—caused by going barefoot on red clay soil, whose minerals irritate the lower lymphatic system in the legs—or lymphatic filariasis (LF), a disease triggered by parasitic worms. Periodic communal foot washing helped those who couldn't reach their own feet and reinforced good hygienic practice, while offering emotional support and a place to share information.

I had arrived at Merawi with a half dozen END Fund donors and board members. Part of my work is connecting people who have resources with people who do not, and doing that in a meaningful and respectful way. The END Fund is a significant investor in Ethiopia's program for neglected tropical diseases (NTDs), which includes all five diseases on our hit list. Over the course of a week, the donors observed a trachomatous trichiasis (TT) surgery, helped at a school-based mass drug administration (MDA) for intestinal worms and schistosomiasis, talked to lab scientists conducting research on river blindness and black flies, met representatives from Ethiopia's deeply committed Federal Ministry of Health, and traveled to Merawi to see the foot washing. One man, Mitku Mengistu, who has elephantiasis in both legs, spoke to us through a translator:

> I used to work as a farmer. I used to be a very good farmer. There was no farmer like me. I used to have a lot of land. I got married with my wife. I have one female and one male child. Soon after, my leg became sick. . . . My leg got hurt. I tried to fix it by knife and brought a black blood from inside. I didn't go to church and get holy water, and soon after the disease expanded to another leg of mine. I felt sick, and it made me lie down for three months. My skin started to peel up, and it became a wounded body. . . . It felt so bad. It had a very bad pain. I stayed home and didn't have anything to give my wife, so she left me. . . . It smelled bad, so people wouldn't approach me. I was afraid and felt shame to approach people.

When we arrived—with no plan to participate—we were welcomed and given an overview of the foot washing by the International Orthodox Christian Charities (IOCC), which was organizing the event. "Who's going to wash feet?" I asked. "Do you think we could help?"

"Are you really interested?" the IOCC rep replied. He was so enthusiastic—they could use some extra hands, the patients would be thrilled—that I asked him to double-check with others. I didn't want to be seen as interloping.

We knelt on straw-covered dirt. Before me, an elderly man with a close-trimmed white beard sat on a bench, a green and blue wrap around his shoulders, holding a long umbrella sheathed in an orange plaid sleeve. His right calf was twice as big as his left. Tough, swollen skin rendered the bones in his feet invisible. On his right foot, the toes were chunky, crammed against each other with indentations where the nails had fallen off. The IOCC rep came around with pink plastic basins, water, and little bars of soap.

I nodded, eyebrows raised, at the man before me. Yes? Okay to begin?

The man nodded. Yes, begin.

■ ■ ■

"I think the first time I was aware of the impact that LF had on a person's livelihood, I was in Léogâne [in Haiti]," said Dr. Patrick Lammie, recalling an early moment in his long career at the Centers for Disease Control and Prevention (CDC).

> I was looking across an empty lot several blocks away. I could see somebody walking, but I could only see the person from the waist up. There was an enormous effort involved in moving forward. There was labor in picking up one foot and, after, the other. Watching him for a moment, I realized that I knew who the patient was. It was a man who was horribly affected by bilateral elephantiasis [of his legs]. Any time I had seen him before, it was always in a clinic, when he would have been sitting in a chair. His life had been irreversibly changed by the development of elephantiasis as a fairly young boy. He had been ostracized. He had had to quit school. Getting along in society was a big challenge for him.

Lymphatic filariasis is transmitted by a mosquito bite. Once inside the host, the filariae (worms) live in the vessels of the lymphatic system, the body's central immune defense mechanism.

Adult worms survive six to eight years, producing millions of microfilariae, which can be transferred to another host by a subsequent mosquito bite. The filariae often damage lymph vessels, causing lymphedema, but sometimes the infection occurs without obstruction—one of LF's puzzles. For many years, studying the disease presented more questions than answers, a gap that allowed some people to assume that LF was a kind of divine punishment. Moreover, until the 1990s, even the most advanced diagnostics meant taking people's blood at night, often between 10 p.m. and 2 a.m. "That was the best time to get the microfilariae in the blood," explained Dr. Mwele Malecela, who started her career working on LF at Tanzania's National Institute for Medical Research. "Just getting people to come out at night was very difficult. People would wonder, 'Why do you want our blood at night? What kind of sorcery, witchcraft, is this?' And then they would ask, 'So what are you going to do for me?' That was the hardest part of my work at that time, because I felt like, this is so sad that we can't do very much."

"We'd go out and do the bleeding once it got dark," Pat Lammie said. "It seemed like 100 degrees, with bugs all over the place—they were drawn by the lights. These night bleeds, there's a lot of drama." He described the bleeds in Haiti as "street theater." Dancing and music sometimes spontaneously arose among the crowd gathered to watch the scientists.

"You might find a thousand microfilariae per milliliter of blood at midnight and zero at noon," said Dr. David Addiss, whose path toward working in global health began when the medical missionary Dan Fountain stayed with his family in New Jersey. Fountain was an American surgeon working in what was then the Belgian Congo. "Fountain realized after several years that he was taking people to surgery for the same condition, over and over again," Addiss said. "He went to Johns Hopkins University to get a master's in public health and became one of the pioneers of primary health care in Africa. I didn't know all the details when I was 9 years old, but I knew he was an amazing guy who I wanted to grow up to be like."

In places where mosquitoes are nocturnal, microfilariae enter the peripheral blood only at night. Where microfilariae go during the day and what signals them to move back and forth remain unknown. "I was impressed by how little we understood about the disease," Addiss said. "We didn't know what caused the lymphedema to progress to elephantiasis. We didn't have a very good drug treatment. We didn't understand some of the transmission dynamics. It was a disease that had been around for thousands of years, and we understood so little. I was fascinated by the epidemiologic questions and also by the beliefs and fears that were related to this disease. There was fear of transmission through witchcraft and other ways of contagious transmission."

Until the 1990s, the going theory was that lymphedemas were a response of the immune system and that progression of the disease was inevitable. A person would be infected and eventually the immune system would wake up and attack not only the parasite but the lymphatic tissues. But then, why did some people living in LF endemic areas *never* have microfilariae in their blood, while others were infected but never developed the advanced stages of the disease? As scientists tried to understand the disease, their only treatment option was a twelve-day course of diethylcarbamazine (DEC). Addiss recalled one patient:

There was a young Haitian woman, about 16 or 17 years old, who had early-stage lymphedema. I examined her. We took our measurements. I noted from the laboratory records that she had the filarial infection, so I measured out the right amount of DEC tablets, asked her to hold out her hand, and gave her the tablets. She looked at the tablets and looked straight at me, and then threw the tablets on the floor and walked out. She had had that treatment before, and it hadn't worked. She knew that what I was offering her was not going to help. She, in her wisdom, said, "I don't need your medicine. It's not going to do any good for me." What struck me—even though I didn't fully understand it—was the sense of hopelessness and the sense of inevitability of progression, which was being reinforced by our scientific understanding of the disease. We were focused on the infection, and there was a depressive quality, particularly for folks who had advanced disease and were very isolated. The stigma that they had was palpable.

China eliminated LF in the 1980s, using a combination of DEC treatments and distribution of DEC-fortified salt. But in countries with fewer resources, "the reality," Lammie said, "is that salt is a commodity that people will consciously strive to spend the least on that they can. You look at two products and one is twenty cents and the other is forty cents. You can't expect people who are living at the edge of poverty to pay a premium for a commodity, even though it may be a fortified product that's better for them."

■　■　■

In the early 1990s, David Addiss began hearing about a "pioneering physician in Brazil." Dr. Gerusa Dreyer at the Fiocruz Institute rejected the commonly accepted ideas that lymphedema was irreversible and that the acute attacks (recurrent inflammation, often characterized by fever, pain, tenderness, and redness) were caused by the host's immune system fighting its tissue. "She was washing people's legs and claiming that somehow they were getting better," Addiss said. "I met her at some of the early filariasis meetings. She started talking about hygiene and these Hope Clubs that she had. The contrast between what she was describing and what I had experienced was dramatic. I asked her if I could come visit her site. She said, 'First, you have to learn enough Portuguese to talk to the patients, and second, you have to promise to do what you can to bring what I'm doing to Haiti.' "

After about two years, Addiss had enough Portuguese under his belt and the funding to go to Brazil. "The first day I was there, she had what she called a Hope Club," he said.

> It was a cross between a support group and a revival meeting with sixty or seventy people with early-stage lymphedema. There was a lot of singing, a lot of sharing of testimony, a lot of encourage-ment. She would talk about the basic elements of the hygiene and skin care. It reminded me of a church service in the African Amer-ican tradition, with the call-and-response. She was masterful at that. They did a washing demonstration, and people were saying, "You need to do it better there." Everybody was jumping in. It was a very joyful experience, completely in contrast to the very som-ber sense of hopelessness that the patients I was working with in Haiti experienced on a day-to-day basis.

People learned how to wash their swollen limbs, protect open wounds from becoming infected, and massage the limb to stimu-late contraction of the lymphatic vessels. They received informa-tion on elevating the limb whenever possible. The acute attacks, they learned, were infections caused by bacteria entering through wounds or cracks in the skin. Equally important, the Hope Clubs "addressed a lot of the stigma, the sense of isolation, the sense of self-efficacy," Addiss said. "Gerusa studied psychology. She's a great observer of both the human condition and clinical find-ings. These clubs [enabled] people to come together. They were able to identify opportunities for work and engagement. It was a whole society that they hadn't had access to. The sense of isolation and stigma was abolished. The sense of empowerment was really overwhelming."

Despite evidence that Dreyer's patients experienced fewer acute attacks and saw their lymphedemas diminish in size, many working in the LF community were reluctant to accept her work. She was arguing against the pervasive theory that swellings were caused by the immune system, and she was advocating for care as opposed to breaking the transmission cycle.

In 1997, LF was designated as a disease to eliminate by the World Health Assembly (the governing body of WHO, composed of health ministers from member states). Shortly thereafter, a group of researchers met in Australia to discuss what the resolution meant and what the response would look like. "It was crafted not as 'elimination of LF' but as 'elimination as a public health problem,'" said Addiss.

> The terminology that was used was meant to soften this, to say "we may not achieve interrupting transmission," to give us some wiggle room. I did a survey of some of the big names the night before the deliberation started. I said, "Do you think there's any room for morbidity management in this program?" They said, "No way. It will divert resources away from interrupting transmission." I conferred with Gerusa, and the fact that they had worded the resolution as "elimination as a public health problem" provided an opportunity for us, because microfilariae in the blood is not a public health problem. Lymphedema, elephantiasis, hydrocele: those are the public health problems. There was no intention to include morbidity management in the LF program until that moment. Gerusa was so persuasive that by the end of that three-day meeting, the group emerged and then announced to a larger LF meeting that the strategy would have two pillars: interrupting transmission and providing care for those who had the disease.

Dreyer's model of hygiene and skin care has been embedded into LF care in Haiti, India, and many places in Africa, including Merawi. Our foot washing there was not as boisterous as a Hope Club meeting, but there were many smiles, some women wore lipstick, and the toenails on one woman's lymphedemic foot were painted pink.

■ ■ ■

I lathered up my bar of soap and began to wash the elderly man's legs. His skin was leathery, and in parts was as rough as sandpaper. It had no elasticity but was thick and solid, lined with deep, dry crevices. I dunked a piece of gauze in the soapy water and seesawed it between his toes. The gauze, when I pulled it out, was covered with black grime. I rinsed and repeated between each of his toes until the water stayed clear. Then, with a scoop of petroleum jelly, I massaged his legs.

One of the volunteers giving out soap, basins, and clean water was a young woman named Yealemwerk Emshaw. "I am the one who collects the sick ones in the Merawi area," she said through a translator. "They asked me to bring them here, so that is how I am helping them out." Emshaw herself had LF, but thanks to bathing, massage, elevation, and wearing shoes, she was able to work: weighing and grinding food, and helping at the clinic.

> My illness appeared suddenly, for no reason. Back then, I used to walk barefoot. Then, for no reason, my leg started getting bigger. When I put shoes on, it got bigger, then it disappeared. When I used holy water on it, it disappeared. Then, as time went on, my leg kept getting bigger and bigger. But since I have come here and gotten educated about it, it has changed a lot. Now I have been cured. I didn't wash it properly. I wasn't fully taking care of my leg. I was not using Vaseline or moisturizing it, so it kept get-

ting bigger. After I came here, though, I learned how to soak my leg and that cleanliness is important and that I should be wearing shoes. . . .

I teach the patients that they have to be clean. I tell them that if they wash properly and stay clean, with cleanliness they can see a lot of changes. I tell them they should always wear shoes. . . . Some of them don't feel that good though. They don't want to let others find out about their sickness. Some are not willing to go for the checkup. And those that don't follow directions properly, when they don't see any change, they insult me. Some are happy when they see the change in me, that my leg is much better. Some are happy after they come to the clinic. Some of them insult me because they haven't yet recovered, because they haven't taken proper care. They tell me that I used something different to get cured, and they think I get hidden benefits from what I do. . . . Because I am now much better, I want others to feel the same. I want the disease to stop with my generation.

Coming to the clinic was also helpful for Mitku Mengistu, the man with elephantiasis in both legs: "I got a very good lesson. Based on that lesson, I wash my legs and I apply an oil given by the nurse. I am very happy. I hope I will get better soon. After I used the medicine, the injured part started getting better and became smooth. If I am fully normal, I will engage with my work. I love to work, so I will do a very good job. I lead my life by grinding goods. . . . God gave me his blessing and I learned this job. . . . I just live a normal life."

■   ■   ■

In 1999, Mwele Malecela returned to Tanzania after completing her PhD at the London School of Hygiene & Tropical Medicine, where she had pursued the question of why some people could clear the microfilariae while others could not. "What we found," she said, "was that in some people, the host's own immunoglobins were covering the microfilariae and protecting them. Some people are able to camouflage the parasites and hence avoid the host responses, and some people are not. And some people are able to clear parasites immediately, without drugs, without anything."

Her plan to establish a research lab for filariasis and other helminth diseases was abandoned after she received a call from Dr. Eric Ottesen, the project leader of WHO's Filariasis Elimination Program. Ottesen and Dr. C. P. Ramachandran had proposed treating LF with ivermectin, which was already being used against river blindness. Successful pilot treatments had blown open the possibility for LF elimination, and the Mectizan Donation Program was going to expand to include LF. Using MDA against LF was a monumental change. "Instead of treating people 20 at a time, you could do 75,000," Lammie said, recalling Haiti's first MDA, which distributed DEC, not ivermectin (at the time, the Mectizan Donation Program was restricted to Africa).

Around the same time, a new diagnostic tool became available in which filarial antigens—substances that elicit an immune response—could be detected circulating in the host's blood. Developed by Dr. Gary J. Weil, the immunochromatographic card test gave an immediate reading, was more sensitive than blood surveys, and—significantly—could find antigens at any time, ending the need for night bleeds.

In 1998—following the World Health Assembly resolution—SmithKline Beecham (later GlaxoSmithKline) had committed to donating albendazole; when combined with ivermectin, this was a way to eliminate LF. (LF can be treated with either ivermectin or DEC; however, DEC can cause severe complications in people with river blindness and is not used where that disease is endemic.) In time, the LF drug program became the largest preventive chemotherapy program for any of the NTDs. By mid-2018, Cambodia, Cook Islands, Egypt, Maldives, Marshall Islands, Niue, Sri Lanka, Thailand, Togo, Tonga, and Vanuatu eliminated LF as a public health problem, and many more countries reduced infections to such low levels that they no longer required MDA. The number of people needing LF treatment continues to decline dramatically: from 1.4 billion in 2011, to 947 million in 2015, to 856 million in 2016.

When Ottesen called Malecela, a $20 million grant from the relatively new Bill & Melinda Gates Foundation had launched the Global Alliance to Eliminate Lymphatic Filariasis. Some of that money could go to Tanzania. "Why would you want to start a lab when you could make a major contribution?" he asked.

Malecela recalled thinking, "This is what I've wanted to do. I've gone to villages, seen people suffer, and I've had the frustration of not being able to do anything. Now I can come back and work towards eliminating this disease. I was a scientist, not a program manager, but I just became a program manager overnight."

From the start, Tanzania's LF program was based on local ownership. "I had [looked at] this from a totally different angle," Malecela said, "and now I needed to ask questions about how people felt about the disease, how people understood the disease, so that when we started giving the medication, we would give them messages why it was important."

The program launched on October 1, 2000. "That was really a moment of euphoria and at the same time fulfillment," she said. "There was something that could be done. We lined up patients and had our ministers of health wash the patients' feet. It was very important for us to show that this was not contagious. It wasn't a curse. When you had a minister of health kneeling to wash these people's feet, it was very powerful."

To her team, Malecela said, "If we want to do things well, we need to do them as we planned. We can't go all over the country. We can only do one region at a time, and when we do get funds to scale up to more regions, we will. That's how we took it."

The program grew slowly and steadily. When coverage had reached three regions, Malecela called the regional- and district-level leaders together to report on what they were doing. "People felt that this was such an expensive exercise," she said, "but I think it was one of the best things we did. We had the political leadership, we had the district accountant, we had the district medical officer, we had the district executive director, we had the regional commissioners. If they were pointing fingers, we would say, 'The district treasurer is right here. Please tell us why money was not sent.'" Regional commissioners chaired the meetings. Malecela would sit to the side, letting them know that it was their program and their responsibility to make it work. She said:

> One of the things I'm very proud of is building a strong team, and a strong Tanzanian team. A lot of times, people would say, "Maybe you need help." And I would say, "I do need help, but maybe this person needs more skills in a particular area, or maybe you could bring us somebody who would help us for a few months so that we could build capacity, rather than have people come in and basically take over the office." That's something I was very adamant about, and it didn't sit well with a number of people who wanted to bring technical assistants to Tanzania to do the work. For me, it was very important that at the end of the day, this was a fully Tanzania-owned program and that whenever the team needed help they would always ask for it. And that anybody who's collaborating with them would respect them enough to say "How can I help?" and not "This is what I think you need."

Money trickled in. The UK government's Department for International Development gave $12,000. "It was just amazing how

$12,000 could go such a long way," Malecela said, "or, at least, we made it go a long way." A subgrant from Gates Foundation funding sustained the program for five years but was not renewed. At one point, WHO offered the program $25,000 to translate into Swahili WHO's LF manual for village health workers.

> We had our own ten-page manual, which we made specifically so the village health worker, the hospital health worker, whoever read that manual got the same message. We said, "Give us the money to make our ten-page booklet into a nice little book or pamphlet." "No, no, no, no, no. This is the WHO book we're going to give you $25,000 to translate into Swahili." I said, "We're not going to do this. It's not going to work, so we don't want to waste your money. But please give us that money to do something useful." They did not give us the money. That experience made me bolder, that ability to say no when you have absolutely nothing. To say no to $25,000. But then I would go and cry and say, "Oh my God, how am I going to do this?"

Another organization offered the Tanzania program $50,000 for billboard marketing:

> They said, "We have this consultant who's come from Coca-Cola." I said, "For us, the village poetry and the traditional dancers mean so much more than billboards. Can we spend our money doing that?" Their whole concept was based on billboards, on heavy marketing. I said, "If you spend $50,000, how much money am I going to spend on doing the actual delivery?" There was a bit of silence, and I said, "I'd like to do what I know works in my country, and what I know works—I'm not just being stubborn—is poems, is African dance, is the stories. That's what works." I lost that money as well. Partners mean well, but most partners don't know your country as well as you do.

Donated drugs can prevent LF. Washing, massage, and elevation help to manage lymphedema and elephantiasis. But these are
useless against hydroceles, another LF complication. These fluid-
filled sacs, usually in the scrotum, may be the size of an orange or
bigger than a basketball. Some hydroceles are so large and heavy
that in order to walk, men carry their scrotums in a wheelbarrow.
Surgery is the only remedy.

In a hydrocelectomy, the scrotum is cut open and the sac that
contains the fluid is drained and turned inside out or largely removed. It is a safe, quick procedure, performed under local anesthesia, which returns a scrotum to its normal size and shape. The
surgery usually costs less than $100.

LF programs often organize surgical camps, that is, high-vol-
ume, time-restricted events focused on one pathology. The goal
is to operate on many people in a short period of time. The END
Fund has underwritten hundreds of hydrocelectomies in Tanzania, with the Ministry of Health choosing a different high-priority
district to receive the funding each year.

Malecela described the atmosphere of a surgical camp: "After
the surgery, at the holding bay, you would sit and chat, and the
men would tell me how their wives had run away from them,
their children had deserted them. These men were really very
stigmatized. Immediately after they had the operation, it was like
this person was invincible." She told me about a hydrocele surgical
camp in Pangani, a town in northeastern Tanzania:

> One of the camps had this wonderful theater, but no equipment.
> So we brought in the equipment, and we put two operating tables
> in each theater. The beauty of that was, because it was local an-
> esthetic, many men could be operated on. The idea was to spend
> some time in the ward. But we said, "We have 200 people. Where
> are we going to get a ward to put 200 people in?"

What we did was we put 20 people in the ward, and then we'd move them into a holding place. I turned classrooms in the school into a holding place, with mattresses and bed nets. The kids were out of school. I got it cleaned up. The chief medical officer said, "Mwele, on your head be it, if anything happens."

People came in, stayed there for three days. Then we had health workers follow up on the people in the village. If the wound was oozing, the person would be brought back to the hospital. By doing that—involving the village health worker, involving this middle stage of having a holding bay—we only had 2 people with postoperative complications—out of 200. One day, the men called me into the ward, and they said, "We want to do a prayer for you." The whole ward together, at the same time. There were 20 men in the ward, and then people in the holding bay had come in. It was packed. It was what they call a Muslim ummah [community]. I'm Christian, so they said, "Just cover your head." And they blessed me, basically. "We wish for you good life. We wish you happiness." And I just said, "Amen, amen, amen."

CHAPTER FIVE

Worms, Maps, and Money

Neglected tropical diseases may be old, but they are not fixed in place. Parasites ride inside tourists, traders, immigrants, and slaves, and they travel across borders, even to new continents. As long as they find a hospitable climate and means of transmission, they survive. Some NTDs have disappeared from various regions. Trachoma spread among people in overcrowded cities in the United States, but diminished as the standard of living rose, including better sanitation, less cramped dwellings, and greater access to clean water. The slave trade brought river blindness from West Africa to Latin America, but thanks largely to the wide distribution of ivermectin, the disease has been eliminated in Colombia, Ecuador, Guatemala, and Mexico, with cases remaining only in the border zone between Brazil and Venezuela.

Hookworm was also brought to the Americas by the slave trade. The US South's warm climate and moist, loamy soil suited the parasite perfectly. Hookworm larvae live up to a month and can travel as far as four feet through soil and grass, feeding and questing for the bare skin of a human host. Pores and hair follicles are open doors for the microscopic larvae, which slip into the bloodstream and wend their way through body tissues to the lungs, from which they go up the trachea, over the epiglottis, and down the esophagus into the gastrointestinal tract, where they make their home in the small intestine. The hookworm's mouth is ringed with semicircular or jagged blades that enable it to latch onto the intestinal wall, from which the worms suck blood. The female drops thousands of eggs per day, which leave the human body in feces. If the infected person defecates onto soil, the eggs have a good chance of hatching larvae, which then seek out a new patch of human skin to penetrate.

A heavy hookworm load is a disaster for the human host, who loses vital amounts of iron and protein through the blood ingested by the worms. Children's physical growth and cognitive development are stunted, and infected people of all ages experience profound lethargy, which is sometimes misinterpreted as laziness. A yellow complexion (protein deficiency) and a desire to eat clay (iron deficiency) are also signs of a hookworm infection. Guitarist Arthur "Blind" Blake summed up the condition in his 1929 song "Hookworm Blues":

> Hookworm in your body
> And your food don't do you no good . . .
> Dirty old hookworm got into my room
> Causes me to walk, groan and moan . . .
> Never can tell what a hookworm man will do.

With the identification of the hookworm *Necator americanus* in 1902, historians started to see the parasite's role in the Civil War—hookworm debilitated Confederate soldiers and destroyed Union soldiers held at the Andersonville prison—while health officials realized that a hookworm epidemic was running through eleven states from Texas to Maryland. In 1909, the Rockefeller Sanitary Commission for the Eradication of Hookworm Disease (RSC) in the US South was formed as a five-year, $1 million project. John Farley writes in *To Cast Out Disease*, a history of the Rockefeller Foundation's early work in health and medicine, "Before the founding of the WHO in 1948, [the Rockefeller Foundation] was arguably the world's most important agency of public health work." He adds, "Hookworm was where it all started."

The Rockefeller Sanitary Commission began by surveying nine states for hookworm; it found the disease prevalent in approximately 40 percent of all children. Attempts to examine people were not always successful, however; in Northampton County, North Carolina, of the 25,000 people surveyed, 22,480 refused to give a stool sample—perhaps because they were required to put the sample in a box and mail it in. Mobile dispensaries treated infected people with the poison thymol, followed by doses of Epsom salts, repeated weekly until stool samples were parasite-free.

The RSC's main attack, however, was through health education aimed at behavior change. Lectures, articles, comic strips, short silent films, and county fair exhibits taught the public how hookworm was transmitted and how it could be prevented. The RSC urged an end to "soil pollution" (the practice of defecating in fields) and recommended that pit latrines be at least four feet deep so that hookworm larvae could not crawl up and out. Contests and competitions awarded points for privies, nearby clean water, good ventilation, hand-washing facilities, and smallpox and typhoid vaccinations. Because of racism, black students were barred from the essay competition, but all families and schools could complete questionnaires ("Is your house screened . . . and how far away is the hog pen?"), making them eligible for prizes such as $5 US government thrift bonds.

"It should be said immediately that [the RSC's] anti-hookworm goal did not for long envision eradication," said Dr. Norman Stoll of the Rockefeller Institute for Medical Research in a seminal 1946 lecture titled "This Wormy World," which was published in 1947. "Instead it evolved, and campaigning exerted itself mostly in blunting the curse in areas which appeared to have the greatest hookworm loads." Between 1909 and 1914, the RSC tested more than 1 million people and treated more than 440,000.

Over time—decades longer than anticipated—hookworm ceased to be a major public health concern in the US South.* The increased use of farm machinery took many workers out of the fields. People left for jobs in cities. And the standard of living rose, meaning more latrines, shoes, paved roads, and access to clean water. The RSC didn't fulfill its mandate of hookworm eradication, but it did increase the general public's knowledge of disease and sanitation, and it helped lay the foundation of a public health system in the region.

Since that initial hookworm campaign, the Rockefeller Foundation has launched thousands of initiatives around the world. Addressing its mission to "improve the well-being of humanity," the foundation supports projects in health, the arts, education, and innovation. From 1978 to 1988 the foundation sponsored the great neglected diseases of mankind (GND) program, a network of scientists, researchers, and doctors working on widely prevalent, largely ignored diseases, including helminthiases (diseases caused by parasitic worm infections). The GND's charismatic leader, Dr. Ken Warren, pitched the idea to the foundation as creating "a critical mass in this field" by fostering international partnerships and collaboration among lab-based scientists, academics, and field workers. Through the network, Warren served as a mentor for several young scientists who then devoted their prominent careers to pursuing the control and elimination of these diseases.

Around the same time—starting in the 1980s and going into the 1990s—a new paradigm on helminthiases took hold. At its core

---

*In 2017, however, an alarming level of hookworm prevalence was detected in Lowndes County, Alabama (34.5 percent of fifty-five stool samples tested positive for *N. americanus*). The region is marked by widespread poverty, and many people are exposed to raw sewage due to inadequate sanitation systems.

were children and schools. Research brought a greater understanding of the far-reaching impact of carrying parasitic worms during childhood. A direct connection between health, education, and economics became clear. Worm-laden children were more likely to miss or fail school—they were not able physically to attend or they were not able cognitively to learn—and this translated into lower wages and lost potential for the rest of their lives.

Historically, helminthiases, like other NTDs, had not been considered important because they were not big killers. Though usually not lethal, these parasites can dramatically reduce one's quality of life, however. Hookworm, roundworm, and whipworm are the world's most prevalent soil-transmitted helminths (STHs); also called intestinal worms, they infect more than a billion people. Roundworm (*Ascaris*) can cause obstruction of the small intestine. Whipworm (*Trichuris*) lodges in the large intestine, causing dysentery and inflammation of the colon. In the late twentieth century, research showed that despite their low mortality, these diseases place massive constraints on human and economic development.

The cost of treatment is very low. "Deworming" refers to the expulsion of worms, most often using the drugs albendazole or mebendazole against STHs and praziquantel to treat schistosomiasis. Deworming can be performed by distributing drugs via schools, which complements distribution in health centers, and through community-based delivery. Schools provide a ready-made infrastructure and a captive audience of children, and they are usually more numerous than health clinics. The main cost is simply getting the medications to the schools. Teachers can be taught to dose drugs, keep records, and incorporate lessons on the diseases and good sanitation and hygiene practices. Schools are used to treat enrolled schoolchildren, but they are also a community center; unenrolled children can be encouraged to come and receive deworming medicines on health days, leading to high coverage.

School-based deworming also has a spillover effect on siblings and other family members, who are then exposed to a smaller pool of parasitic worms.

In "School Based Health and Nutrition Programs," published in the 2006 edition of *Disease Priorities in Developing Countries*, Dr. Donald A. P. Bundy and his colleagues write:

> The focus of school health and nutrition programs in low-income countries has shifted significantly over the past two decades away from a medical approach that favored elite schools in urban centers and toward an approach that improves health and nutrition for all children, particularly the poor and disadvantaged. This change began in the 1980s, when research showed not only that school health and nutrition programs were important contributors to health outcomes but also that they were essential elements of efforts to improve education access and completion, particularly for the poor.

The first edition of *Disease Control Priorities in Developing Countries* had been published in 1993. In a reflection of the work's roots in the GND, the lead author of the chapter "Helminth Infection" was Ken Warren. In the same year—and drawing on the same data analysis—the World Bank published *Investing in Health*, a landmark report that justified health interventions on economic grounds. "The report specifically uses MDA for STH to show that even a disease with low clinical importance and low mortality could be a major source of morbidity and a constraint on development," Bundy told me. "This was a shocking and controversial point at the time. It is now the basic underpinning of the whole rationale for the focus on NTDs."

Using schools as a platform for the delivery of deworming drugs and education has been a focus through much of Bundy's career, which has included serving as the lead health and education specialist at the World Bank and as a senior advisor on NTDs at the Gates Foundation. "In places where there were no health systems, the school was often the unique structure, the unique institution where you could actually access kids of that age," he said. "Using schools to deliver health became a part of a contribution to human physical, cognitive, and, ultimately, economic development."

In 1990, Don Bundy founded the Partnership for Child Development (PCD) with support from the Rockefeller Foundation, the UN Development Programme, and others. The PCD brought together a wide range of organizations to focus on improving the lives of children. "In 1990 the idea of partnerships was novel," Bundy recalled. "The idea that actually, you mean, we all work together? That was emerging as a new idea. And that it was about child development, which was a turnoff in much of the health community. All health was about mortality and survival, so calling it 'child development' was a very specifically soft message. Both of those messages—a partnership and development, as against a task force and survival—were a deliberate antithesis to the Task Force for Child Survival, for the best of reasons." These reasons included the fact that the Task Force for Child Survival, established in the 1980s by Dr. William H. Foege, was succeeding in keeping more children alive. The issue that remained was the *quality* of their lives.

■ ■ ■

In the late 1990s, the American economist Dr. Michael Kremer returned to Kenya, where he had taught English for a year after college. A friend there was working at Internationaal Christelijk Steunfonds Africa (ICS), a Dutch NGO focused on improving education, and had been assigned to choose seven new schools to implement ICS's child sponsorship program. "I suggested that they could start out with a larger set of schools and then choose randomly within that to evaluate the impact of the program," said Kremer. The leadership at ICS agreed and began experimenting with various classroom changes, including more textbooks and more teachers. "Some things didn't work, some things worked, some things had mixed results." Influenced by *Investing in Health*, Kremer suggested deworming. ICS implemented the treatment in seventy-five schools, which were put in geographic and alphabetical order and then divided into three groups.

"In the first year, the group 1 schools got dewormed," Kremer said. "In the second year, the group 2 schools got dewormed with group 1. By the fourth year, the third group was phased in. By comparing the outcomes in the different groups, you could be relatively confident that that was due to the difference of deworming, rather than anything else."

Of all the programs ICS had implemented, deworming had the lowest price and the greatest effect. School attendance rose by 25 percent. The cost per additional year of school participation was US$3.50.

The data, published by Edward Miguel and Michael Kremer in *Econometrica* in 2004, came at an opportune moment for Dr. Simon Brooker, a professor of epidemiology at the London School of Hygiene & Tropical Medicine, who was working at the Kenya Medical Research Institute (KEMRI). "My interest was around trying to increase the evidence base around rational, cost-effective NTD programs," said Brooker. His goal was to help the sponsors of programs make "smarter, more data-driven" decisions.

"A large area of our early work was to investigate the geographical distribution of these diseases, understand the factors that influence their distribution, identify the areas and estimate the population requiring treatment and drug needs, and, crucially, help target treatment to areas of greatest need," he said. The low cost and high impact of drugs meant nothing if they weren't going to the places where people needed them, or if they were being wasted by going to places where people didn't need them. "I was very interested in mapping," said Brooker. "Here you had these diseases for which we had effective interventions which could be delivered through low-cost platforms, such as schools. But we didn't know where the diseases were, so we weren't able to target treatment according to need."

The mapping gap wasn't due to a lack of research. By the early 2000s, *thousands* of worm surveys had been conducted in Kenya, yet there was not a national program. In one district in western Kenya, for example, 120 surveys had been done—all research, no implementation. Funds in the Ministry of Health's budget, earmarked for a deworming program, went unspent each year. Simon Brooker remarked:

> Kenya is a very environmentally varied country: deserts, snow-capped mountains, forests, and savannas. We know from the biology of these worms that their ability to survive in different environments varies. One of the early pieces of research that we did was trying to show how you can link the distribution of these worms with environmental factors, using data derived from satellites to provide estimates of such variables as temperature, vegetation, and humidity. First, we sought to collate quality surveys identified from structured searches of the literature into a standardized database, according to specific inclusion criteria. Second, we geolocated the surveys to help develop maps. Finally, we used statistical modeling to predict infection levels in the areas without data.

Brooker recalled a discussion with an administrator from a northwestern region of Kenya:

> He was quite adamant that any deworming program should be extended to his district, for political reasons. We presented this map

that we'd developed, and we said, "Actually, there's not a problem of worms here, so your district does not need to be dewormed, and you can use your resources to address other health problems." That showed to the government that you could have a national program but one which was targeted to the areas in greatest need. The developed maps were a main reason why the Kenya program was initiated along the coast and in western Kenya. This approach ensured (a) efficient allocation of scarce resources, and (b) the program has the largest impact by targeting the populations in greatest need.

While Simon Brooker was assembling data for Kenya and the rest of Africa, the results of Miguel and Kremer's deworming study were published, joining a growing body of research that framed deworming as an issue of economics and education as much as health. Multiple studies found that children not only spent more days in school, but their ability to learn improved: those who were less than a year old when they were dewormed had cognitive gains comparable to almost a year of schooling; the siblings and neighbors of children who were dewormed also benefited. Some years later, Miguel and Kremer followed up with the children in their original study. Those who had been dewormed were earning more money because they had stayed in school longer and could work longer hours.

The Deworm the World Initiative was launched in 2007 by Michael Kremer, with support from the PCD and Innovations for Poverty Action. Its premises are that parasitic worms greatly reduce a child's potential for learning, growing, and, later, earning money; deworming drugs are available, safe, and inexpensive; and schools provide an infrastructure for drug distribution that yields high coverage when school attendance is sufficiently high. Basically, the world would be a better place if all children at risk of parasitic worms were dewormed at least once per year.

Since its beginning, Deworm the World—now an initiative of Evidence Action, an organization focused on scaling up evidenced-based global health and development interventions—has provided technical assistance to governments in Ethiopia, India, Kenya, Nigeria, Pakistan, and Vietnam to implement large-scale, school-based deworming programs, supporting treatment for hundreds of millions of children. Evidence Action is part of a broad coalition of organizations and countries that see deworming children as a global priority. According to WHO, in 2016 over 60 percent of more than 800 million children in need of treatment globally actually received the medicines they needed, a number that has steadily climbed from under 20 percent in 2008. About half of 100 million children requiring treatment for schistosomiasis were treated in 2016, up from about 15 percent in 2011. There has been great progress, but many children are still not being reached.

■ ■ ■

In the 1920s, Watson Rankin, secretary of the North Carolina State Board of Health, encouraged by leaders of the International Health Board (successor to the RSC), publicized the "unit costs" and "cost equivalents" of the hookworm campaign. Arbitrarily, Rankin decided that every educational lecture returned ten cents per person to the community, every newspaper article returned $5, and every privy $5. Wanting to foster a competitive spirit, he also altered health forms so that counties in his state could be ranked according to "earnings per dollar invested." Thankfully, Rankin would have a hard time fabricating data in today's global health environment and particularly within the NTD community, which is a close-knit and highly connected group. People from around the world share and publish their data, meet at conferences, and work together on problems that no one could solve on their own. Data transparency is fundamental. Websites like the Global Atlas of

Trachoma and the Global Atlas of Helminth Infections help make this possible. The site for helminth infections takes its URL from the title of Norman Stoll's lecture: www.thiswormyworld.org. Both sites are open access, meaning anyone can obtain the raw data.

"This is something I've always felt very strongly about: that data are really a public good," said Simon Brooker, who was involved in the creation of both sites and later became a senior program officer at the Gates Foundation. One provision of receiving a grant from Gates—and an increasing number of other foundations—is that any ensuing publication is open access. Not only does this promote transparency, it helps ensure that really good data don't become buried treasure, left behind on a computer when a researcher changes jobs or moves on to another project. Open access also helps ensure that program decisions and commitments are based on facts. Brooker said:

> [With the Global Atlas of Helminth Infections,] what we wanted to do was, first, compile all of the available data that went through some sort of quality control procedure into a single database, to develop maps, and then make the data and maps publicly available. In doing so, we hoped to create a resource—a global public good—which policy makers and national programs would use to guide their decision-making. All too often, public health decisions were not—and are still not—based on data, but rather on opinion and precedent. We sought to change this by increasing access to data and improving the use of data for decision-making.

In the mid-2000s, Brooker and Dr. Narcis Kabatereine from the Uganda Ministry of Health developed a new rapid mapping method for schistosomiasis. Compared to STHs, schistosomiasis has a very localized distribution, meaning that treatment may need to be targeted on a school-by-school or subdistrict basis, rather than by district. Brooker and Kabatereine based their rapid mapping method on lot quality assurance sampling, a practice that originated in manufacturing. Rather than test every product manufactured, a few items from a batch (or lot) are examined. On a production line, two defects in a given lot might be within the acceptable margin of error, but greater than two would mean pulling the entire lot. "This was applied in the 1990s to validating reported vaccination coverage, to be able to quickly do surveys to see whether you've got sufficiently high vaccination coverage," Brooker said. "It had been used in other areas, but it hadn't been applied to NTDs. Through a combination of computer simulations and field studies, we showed that if you sampled just fifteen children in every school, that was sufficient to decide whether you needed to intervene. If you had more than seven [children infected with schistosome parasites], that indicated that it was greater than 50 percent prevalence. It didn't give you a reliable estimate of infection prevalence, but provided rapid mapping data to guide deworming."

A reluctance to map persisted as recently as the early 2000s. Brooker recalled a conversation with a senior WHO official. "Categorically they said, 'There's no point mapping. We don't need to map. We just need to treat everywhere.' When we really started to do mapping and promote the idea of mapping, there was a lot of resistance. The argument went like this: the tablets are really cheap, and we know that schools are a great delivery system. Why would we spend money on doing surveys? It was felt it would divert resources from the main task at hand, which obviously is providing treatment."

In 1999, Don Bundy had asked Brooker and his colleagues to map worms and other health problems among schoolchildren in Chad, where at least thirty years had passed since the last survey. The budget was $50,000. Brooker proposed using satellite imagery to develop ecological zones, which would give the surveyors a broad idea of the expected distribution of worms.

"We didn't go to the north because that's the Sahara Desert," he said. "At the time, in the east, it was unsafe due to civil strife. But we divided the other areas into these ecological zones and sampled schools from each zone to be surveyed and in doing so provided a representative distribution of STH and schistosomiasis." The goal was "to generate good-quality evidence to make decisions. We were not trying to precisely estimate prevalence." Rather, they sought to use low-cost data to answer the simple question: Where does the country need to implement deworming? The result led to a much more targeted, effective deworming program. Fewer people, simpler logistics, and less money were needed in the long term, and efforts were focused on areas with the highest burden of disease.

■　■　■

In 2006, Elie Hassenfeld and Holden Karnofsky, two young hedge-fund analysts, wanted to figure out where they could donate to charity in order to have the greatest impact—the most bang for each buck. "We expected that we'd go to the internet and search for a high-impact charity, and we'd find really great information about where to give," recalled Hassenfeld. "But instead of finding great information, we found almost nothing that was helping us make great giving decisions. There was very little helpful, evidence-backed information about which charities were doing the most good."

Hassenfeld, Karnofsky, and six colleagues started meeting bi-weekly. "We decided that we'd each pick a cause, research that cause, and then we'd pool our results and give donations by the end of 2006." Hassenfeld's cause was clean water in Africa. Twenty dollars would provide a child with clean water for life, the water charities assured him. "I was like, 'That's amazing. Now, just help me understand how you arrived at that calculation. Where are the budgets, and what did you do with the money, and where did it go?'" The organizations would send glossy annual reports with colorful pictures, but either couldn't or wouldn't give out their data. "There was absolutely no substantive information about the programs or how well they were working," Hassenfeld said. "Holden called up an organization. He just wanted to know how much money they spent in each of the countries that they had worked in. We had an idea—if you knew what country they were working in, you could look at the burden of disease and do some sort of back-of-the-envelope calculation of cost-effectiveness. The fact that he asked those questions made the organization think he was a spy for a separate competitor organization, because why else would any donor ever ask these questions?"

By mid-2007, what had started as a side project became all-consuming. "I remember being up late on a Saturday night," Hassenfeld said, "and it's three in the morning, and I was reading academic papers about diarrhea in Africa. I felt like I found the subject matter that I was incredibly passionate about. It was that combination: the passion for the research and the recognition that this information really wasn't out there." Hassenfeld and Karnofsky quit their jobs at the hedge fund to launch GiveWell, a "nonprofit dedicated to finding outstanding giving opportunities and publishing the full details of our analysis to help our donors decide where to give" (according to its website). Its transparency extends to a section online titled "Our Mistakes."

GiveWell starts with an intervention and then asks, how much evidence is there that it works? How cost-effective is it? Who is implementing that program? "Our idea was that we wanted there to be absolutely no friction for a donor who wanted to assess whether our research was worth following," Hassenfeld said.

"They can just use our research for free, if that's what they choose to do, and never talk to us at all."

Early on, Hassenfeld and Karnofsky were advised to look at deworming for schistosomiasis and intestinal worms. They reviewed the initial and follow-up studies by Michael Kremer and Ted Miguel, which "really made deworming look to us like an incredibly strong, very cost-effective intervention," Hassenfeld said. "It's so cheap to treat a child with deworming, and then you can potentially have this very long-term, very large effect on people's income, presumably driven—we don't really know the mechanism—but presumably driven by improvements in schooling or cognitive development or physical development, that allows people to earn more money."

GiveWell's recommendation of deworming is tempered, however. GiveWell believes that the evidence for the short-term benefits of deworming is complicated, but the cheapness of the intervention and the impact seen in the follow-up studies on the treated children's incomes later in life make deworming one of the most cost-effective interventions GiveWell has found. Elie Hassenfeld said:

> I still think the overall picture is far from clear. There's evidence of short-term effects from deworming treatments when the infections are extremely serious. But when the infections are less intensive, there's a big debate about what level and what types of effects you can expect. . . . Our current view is that deworming is really one of the best bets for people who are interested in using money to increase development worldwide. We think it's far from certain because the evidence is, in many ways, very complicated. But deworming is so cheap and the organizations that we recommend that implement this program do their work in a very high-quality way. It's the combination of the evidence, the cost-effectiveness,

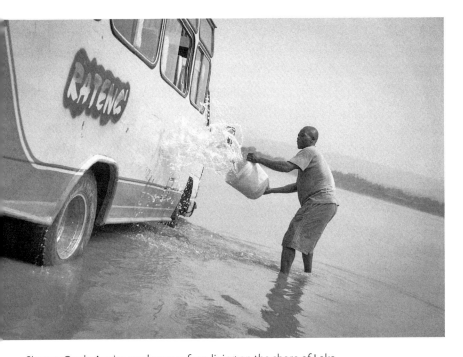

Simeon Ogola Aquiro washes cars for a living on the shore of Lake Victoria near Kisumu, Kenya. Many people whose lives depend on the lake—like fishers and car washers—are exposed daily to the parasites that cause schistosomiasis, which, without treatment, can result in serious illness and even death. Mo Scarpelli/END Fund

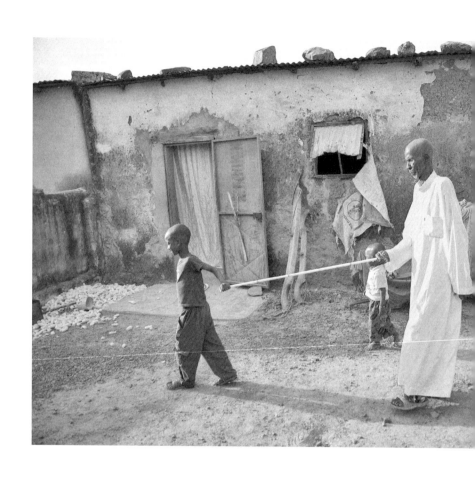

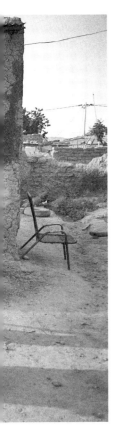

Moce, which means "grandfather" in Bambara, has lived with river blindness for more than thirty years. Treatment in his home country of Mali started as aerial spraying of pesticide by helicopter to kill the black flies that carry the vector for this disease; by 1987 Mali had transitioned to treatment with the newly discovered medicine ivermectin. This treatment means that the younger generations won't have to face the disabling effects of this disease. Jonathan Olinger and Lindsay Branham of Discover the Journey / END Fund

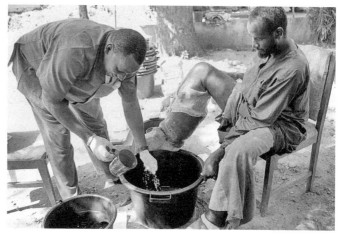

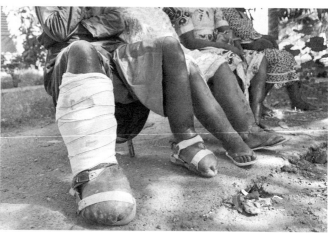

Bani has an advanced stage of lymphatic filariasis, which can manifest as elephantiasis of the lower extremities. He helps to organize and is the spokesperson for a patient support group that meets regularly to learn how to care for their condition and to receive foot washings and wound treatment. More than a billion people are at risk for lymphatic filariasis, and millions have various forms of the advanced conditions, which require special care or surgery. Jonathan Olinger and Lindsay Branham of Discover the Journey/END Fund

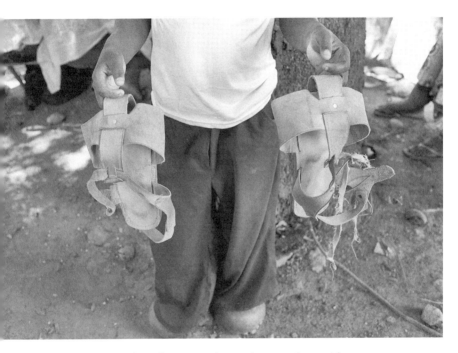

In addition to needing deep cleansing and wound care, patients with elephantiasis, like Oumar, often use special shoes like these to ensure they can remain mobile. Jonathan Olinger and Lindsay Branham of Discover the Journey / END Fund

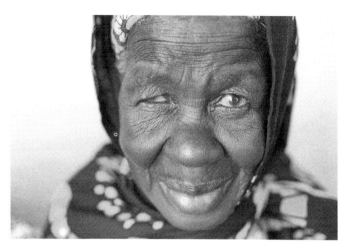

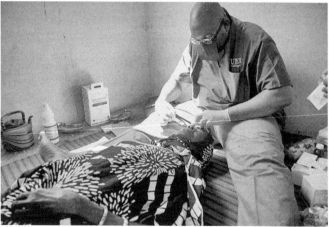

Trachoma is the most common infectious cause of blindness in the world. Nieba shows the telltale symptom of an opaque cornea, which comes after many years of multiple, painful trachoma infections. The ophthalmic nurse performed a twenty-minute surgery, with local anesthesia, to stop her progression toward blindness. Jonathan Olinger and Lindsay Branham of Discover the Journey / END Fund

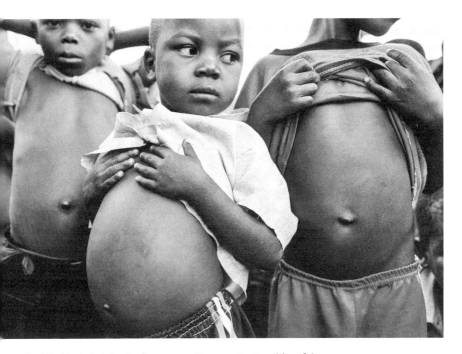

On Idjwi in Lake Kivu in the eastern Democratic Republic of the Congo, the remote island's first-ever mass deworming program was launched in 2015. More than 84 percent of children and adults there were found to have one or more neglected tropical diseases, with intestinal worms the most common. One of the practices conducted by traditional healers to try to remediate the swollen bellies caused by worms and malnutrition was to make small cuts with razor blades on the children's stomachs, which sometimes led to infection or worse.
Mo Scarpelli/END Fund

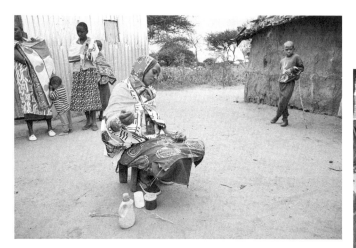

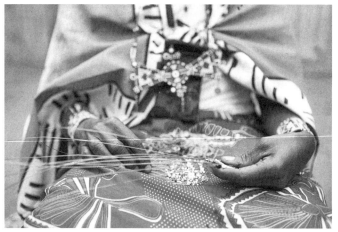

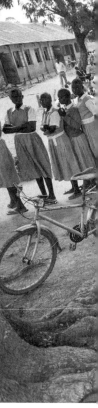

Susan, a member of the Maasai community in Kenya, had suffered from trachomatous trichiasis, but she had a successful twenty-minute surgery to stop her progression to blindness. She now talks to people in her community, who might be nervous about getting the surgery, to share her experience of the process and its benefits. For Susan, it has meant that she can continue her business making and selling beaded traditional jewelry. Mo Scarpelli / END Fund

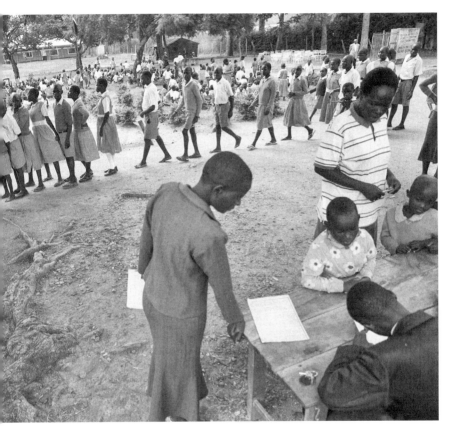

School-based deworming days, like this one in Bungoma, Kenya, are often festive events. Hundreds of children line up in the schoolyard to watch skits from the school hygiene club, take deworming medicines, and learn about the impact of tropical diseases in their local communities. Mo Scarpelli / END Fund

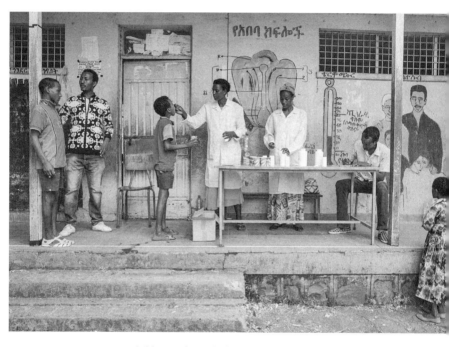

Every child goes through the basic steps seen here at a school-based mass drug administration in Merawi, Ethiopia. Students are measured for height, which determines how many pills they will need to take to treat each disease. Community health workers then give the medicines—in this case, albendazole for intestinal worms and praziquantel for schistosomiasis—to each child, and the data are logged into a treatment register. Mo Scarpelli / END Fund

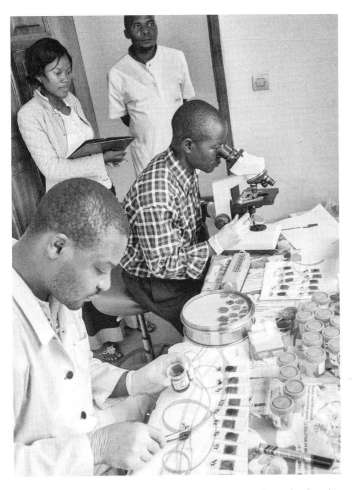

A temporary mapping station was set up in 2015 on Idjwi Island in the eastern Democratic Republic of Congo, where technicians counted the number of eggs in stool samples. Higher numbers of eggs indicate the presence of more intestinal worms and a greater chance for illness. Saskia Keeley / END Fund

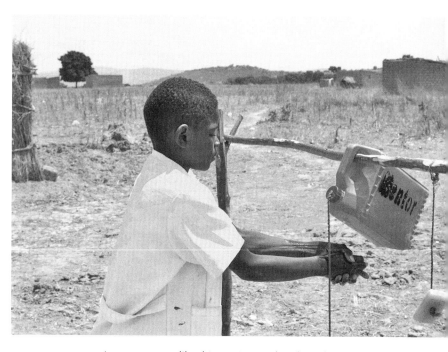

In remote areas like this one in Angola, where there is no running water in schools or homes, a tippy tap is a practical, low-tech hand-washing station. Kids and adults are able to wash their hands and face with a small amount of dripping water. This simple intervention dramatically improves hygiene and therefore health, reducing both trachoma and intestinal worm infections. MENTOR/Dubai Cares

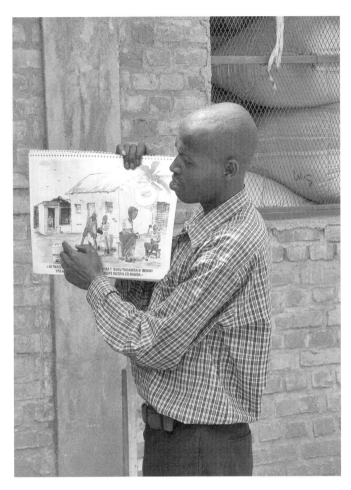

A government health worker in Rutana, Burundi, provides education on NTD prevention as part of a post-treatment strategy. The importance of using latrines and of washing hands before preparing food is emphasized to prevent the spread of intestinal worms. James Porter / END Fund

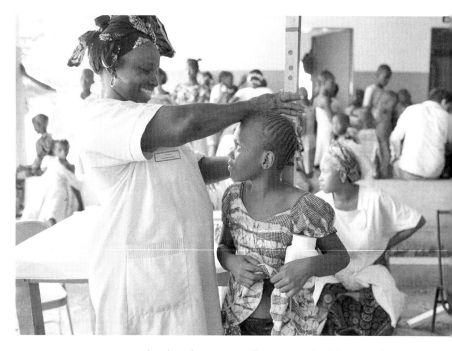

Dose poles show how many pills a person should receive for each medicine during a mass drug administration. These poles can be made of wood, as shown here; they can be a piece of folded paper taped to a wall; or they can be a length of fabric that fits easily into a community health worker's bag. This child will receive one albendazole pill (indicated by the top dot) and three ivermectin pills (the three lower dots). Jonathan Olinger and Lindsay Branham of Discover the Journey / END Fund and the organizations that has led us to recommend deworming for so many years.

This measured view of deworming is shared by William MacAskill, cofounder and president of Giving What We Can (GWWC), whose members pledge to donate 10 percent of their earnings and actively research and debate which organizations to give to. MacAskill helped launch the effective altruism (EA) movement, which is dedicated to putting money, time, and resources where they can do as much good as possible. Both GWWC and EA have recommended deworming for its *expected* impact. Hassenfeld elaborated on this point: "People assume that kids who are being dewormed have very obvious clinical manifestations of disease. So, one challenge that we've had is helping people understand what this intervention [deworming] is. Another challenge that we've faced is how we talk about the evidence. . . . On balance, there's this uncertainty and there's some risk, but once you take that into account, we think it's one of the best giving opportunities we know of."

Deworming programs run by Evidence Action, the END Fund, Schistosomiasis Control Initiative, and Sightsavers are among GiveWell's "top charities," which also include organizations that focus on malaria, vitamin A supplementation, loans, and direct cash transfers. Since its founding, GiveWell has moved more than $350 million, via more than 50,000 donors, to the charities it recommends.

Another organization offering a rational approach to philanthropy is the Copenhagen Consensus Center, which compares the costs and benefits of a range of development proposals—from education to nutrition to air quality. In 2010, Copenhagen Consensus listed deworming as the sixth most effective action a philanthropist could support. Its founder and director, Bjørn Lomborg, explained:

If you're going to spend your own money, of course you look at "what am I going to get for my money at one place compared to other places?" But we're a little uncomfortable about doing this in the space of development. Intellectually it makes a lot of sense, but emotionally it feels really wrong. We don't want to take away resources from things that feel good. But the reality is, if you spend money on things that do fairly little good, that's money you can't spend on stuff that could do an amazing amount of good. We should have that conversation, so that the decision where to spend money is not predominantly focused on who is best able to capture the public imagination and the public purse, which often comes down to who has the most compelling story. A lot of prioritization comes down to who has the most crying kids or the cutest animals or the best PR groups, and you can see why that would be the case, but truly that's not how it should be.

Given that today almost all of the medicines to treat the most prevalent NTDs are donated by pharmaceutical companies, the main cost to countries' health systems and their partners is delivery. Early estimates placed this at about fifty cents per person per year. A deeper dive into these numbers suggests that this is a helpful starting place, but in some cases—in the most rural and hard-to-reach places with no previous treatment history—the cost can run upward of a dollar. In places with greater efficiency and integrated treatment, the cost can be less than twenty cents per person per year. In "An Investment Case for Ending Neglected Tropical Diseases" (2016), Christopher Fitzpatrick and his colleagues write: "The net benefit to affected individuals is about US$25 for every dollar . . . invested by public and philanthropic funders between 1990 and 2030—a 30 percent annualized rate of return."

Treating NTDs is a best buy for global health. It is inexpensive and yields many kinds of return: educational, medical, financial, and moral. A central premise of the Rockefeller Sanitary Commission was that it was making an *investment*, not performing charity. "The time will come when [the people] will demand clear-cut evidence of [the county health work's] value just as stockholders in a company demand dividends on investments," wrote the state director of the Sanitary Commission for North Carolina and associate director of the International Health Board. Forty cents per head would save 300–500 lives and improve the health of 6,000–7,000 people per year, stated a March 1919 editorial in the *Raleigh News and Observer*, explaining the North Carolina law requiring households to install a latrine or pay a fine.

"School enrollment, regular school attendance, and literacy increased markedly in counties that had previously suffered from high rates of hookworm infection," notes Hoyt Bleakley in a 2007 paper in which he analyzes the RSC survey and treatment data as well as wage and salary information from the 1940 US Census. "Children with more exposure to the campaign, by being born later and in a state with greater treatment intensity, [were] more likely to be literate and earn higher incomes as adults," Bleakley writes. "There is indeed evidence of an increase in the return to schooling as a result of the intervention," and "the intervention had the effect that children attended school more intensively."

Bleakley also cites a Hardin County, Texas, newspaper, which commended the county commissioners for designating $300 for the operational expenses of five hookworm dispensaries. "According to the editorial, '300 dollars was never spent for a better purpose.'"

CHAPTER SIX

A New Normal

"You see the urine, very red in color," said Dr. Chinyelu Ekwunife, professor of parasitology at Nnamdi Azikiwe University, who has studied and fought schistosomiasis in Nigeria for more than a decade. "You talk with them, 'What is this?' They say it's meant to live with them. It's part of life. By the time you are 12 or 13 years old, you must pass blood in your urine. It's a part of growing up."

In fact, blood in the urine—hematuria—is a common early sign of urogenital schistosomiasis, a disease also known as bilharzia or snail fever. In some communities, the onset of hematuria in adolescent boys is seen as male menstruation, a sign of puberty. It is considered normal, as are many hallmarks of long-term infections with NTDs: opaque eyes (blinded by trachoma or river blindness); skin lacking pigment and elasticity, marked by worm-filled nodules and relentless itching (evidence of onchocerca skin disease); or a distended abdomen (indicating long parasitic worms living in a person's intestine). When so many people look and feel the same, the sickness, discomfort, and deformities are part of everyday life.

"People actually don't know they can feel a lot better," said Dr. Dirk Engels, a Belgian tropical medicine physician who directed the NTD program at WHO's headquarters in Geneva from 2014 to 2017. "It is only when you carry out large-scale treatment for the parasites they are chronically infected with that they realize how bad they have been. With the result that, the next time they see you, they run after your car for more treatment. Many of us who have worked in the field have experienced that. And it has been a great encouragement for us to take the solution to scale during the rest of our careers."

Until very recently, NTDs have been ignored not just by people at risk for the diseases but by doctors and other medical professionals, whose priorities since the late twentieth century have been the big killers: HIV/AIDS, tuberculosis, malaria, vaccine-preventable childhood diseases like polio, pneumonia, and diarrheal diseases. "It was just normal to have children with intestinal worms," said Dr. Corine Karema, former director of the Malaria and Other Parasitic Diseases Division at the Rwanda Biomedical Center. *If* a child was brought to a clinic and *if* a nurse thought to test for intestinal worms or schistosomiasis and *if* someone at the clinic had the training to diagnose using the Kato-Katz test (counting worm eggs in a stool sample under a microscope), *then* the child would receive medicine to expel the worms. Given the obstacles, these dewormings were rare. In 2005, Rwanda launched a maternal and child health week, which included deworming for children under 5 years old, but worms in adolescents and adults still were "not taken as a public health problem," Karema said.

"I've seen patients die from schistosomiasis," said Engels. He spent his early career in rural Zambia, Senegal, Rwanda, and Zimbabwe. Working in Burundi, where schistosomiasis cases had been located around a mountain lake in the north, Engels went to the nuns at a mission hospital nearby.

"We don't have that disease here," he recalled a nun saying.

"I said, 'Sister, can I propose something? You see that line out there, waiting for the consultations? Let's ask for a stool examination of each of them, and then let's look together, right?'"

"'It's just to please you,' she said, 'because I'm convinced we don't have that disease here.'"

"We did that, and one-third of those in the line had schisto. I called the lab technician and I said, 'Why didn't you report that?' He said, 'I didn't know it was important, because the sister hadn't told me that this was important.'"

■ ■ ■

At conferences and meetings, I've asked public health professionals, "When did you first encounter NTDs?"

"Not that long ago," many of them answered, despite years working in Africa. Then they clarified that they had seen *signs* of the diseases—bellies distended with intestinal parasites, people struggling to walk due to elephantiasis of the legs—but not *treatment*. Given the other priorities, NTDs weren't screened for and didn't qualify as a top public health concern.

Even Dr. Matshidiso Moeti, the director of WHO's Regional Office for Africa, acknowledged, "My personal involvement in NTDs has been very recent." Moeti's medical education is rooted in her childhood in South Africa; both of her parents were doctors, and their practice was in a room built as an addition off the back of their house to serve the poor community in their township. "As a child, I used to see this traffic of people coming in to see my parents, so I was very much used to seeing sick people, pregnant mothers, and if my parents weren't in the surgery they were out doing house calls." Her father was part of the smallpox commission, going door to door looking for cases. From ongoing family conversations about maternal and child health, tuberculosis, and smallpox, young Moeti "got absorbed" into medicine and public health.

"Did you know about NTDs as a child?" I asked her. "Did you get dewormed?"

"No."

"Did you know people had bilharzia?"

"Actually not," she said. "Isn't that strange?"

Moeti's early career in Botswana took her from clinical work at a district hospital during the pretreatment days of HIV/AIDS to running the hospital's tuberculosis ward to directing the country's communicable diseases control program. "I have to acknowledge we were hardly thinking about neglected tropical diseases," she said. "I was aware in a certain way that somewhere in the central district of Botswana there's this problem, and schistosomiasis up in the northwest, where there's water and rivers. As for deworming: never thought about it."

Working on HIV/AIDS was "one of the most notable, difficult, exciting, and challenging experiences of my whole career," she said, "because it was in those early days of HIV/AIDS. No treatment was available. We used to keep a secret register of the people who tested positive because of all the stigma." She moved to Zambia for a job at UNICEF. "Zambia was doing radical health reform programming," she recalled. "But NTDs? No. Not even deworming. I'm trying to recall if one was aware of the need, the importance, the usefulness of deworming school kids." She thought for a moment. "No."

Years later, Moeti was introduced to an NTD program by chance. While working as the WHO representative in Malawi, she received a call from Dr. Uche Amazigo, director of the African Programme for Onchocerciasis Control (APOC). Amazigo was calling because Malawi was late reporting on its APOC funding and risked not receiving the next round. Could someone chase down the report? The year was 2006. After decades in medicine and public health, Moeti learned of the river blindness program because the director of APOC needed help getting a report.

How did these diseases elude attention for so long?

On the one hand, the diseases are considered "part of life." The signs and symptoms of NTDs are obvious—and ignored. On the other hand, people carrying the diseases try to make themselves unseen. Stigmatized, they reduce their time in public, at school, or at work. "Family members avoid them, marginalize them," said Dr. Seifu Tirfie, the country representative for Ethiopia at International Orthodox Christian Charities. "Most of them choose to go to churches, monasteries. Even there, they might have difficulties because . . . the bacterial infection [of lymphatic filariasis] might bring some really bad smell, so people push them out."

The modern NTD effort includes tangible solutions—pills, surgeries, tippy taps, bed nets—as well as questions without simple answers. Cleanliness is integral to trachoma prevention, but how far must villagers walk to reach a clean water source? Swallowing a pill for schistosomiasis on an empty stomach may cause a child to vomit, but what if she hasn't eaten recently? Does she have access to adequate food? If NTDs are a normal part of life, what is normal? Must "normal" mean "inevitable"?

■ ■ ■

The parasite responsible for schistosomiasis hides in plain sight inside its human host. "It lives in the blood vessel and is not detected," said Professor Alan Fenwick, who founded the Schistosomiasis Control Initiative (SCI) in the Department of Infectious Disease Epidemiology at Imperial College London. "The body's immune system does not kill the worm. The worm somehow manages very quickly to coat itself with human material. It's like a Harry Potter invisibility cloak. The worm is just not recognized."

This disguise partly explains the durability of the schistosome parasite, which has existed for at least 3,000 years. Calcified *Schistosoma haematobium* eggs were found in the kidneys of two Egyptian mummies dating from the Twentieth Dynasty (circa 1000 BCE). *Schistosoma japonicum* eggs dating from 168 BCE were found in a noble woman's remains in China's Hunan Province. This "incredibly clever creature" (according to Fenwick) spends its early life in fresh water, used by people for bathing, washing clothes and utensils, cooking, drinking, and irrigation. People may swim in schistosome-infested water, or it may be a source of income, for example, for fishers.

Snails provide shelter for the schistosome's early development into larvae, which then, using forked tails, swim out in search of human skin. Once inside their new host, the parasites drop their tails and ride through blood vessels until they reach the portal vein of the liver, where adult male and female schistosomes mate. In pairs, they migrate to the blood vessels of either the intestine (*S. mansoni* and *S. japonicum*) or the bladder and reproductive organs (*S. haematobium*). Gorging on hemoglobin, the female produces a daily batch of hundreds of eggs, each with a single spine that is used to drill through blood vessel walls to reach the intestine or bladder, from which they leave the body, carried by feces or urine. When this egg-laden waste is deposited in or near a body of fresh water, new schistosome larvae (miracidia) hatch from the eggs and search for snail hosts—and the next cycle begins.

A nearly universal consequence of schistosomiasis is anemia: hemoglobin is taken by the parasite for food, and there is blood loss when eggs attempting to move through the wall of the bladder or intestine become trapped, rupturing small blood vessels. (This is the blood that appears in urine or feces.) The ruptured blood vessels trigger an inflammatory response that can lead to the stretching and swelling of the ureter, kidneys, or liver. Urine flow can become blocked. Lesions may form on the vulva, vagina, cervix, or uterus. The fallopian tubes or vas deferens can become obstructed, potentially causing impotence, sterility, and miscarriage. Schistosomiasis also makes its hosts more susceptible to other diseases, in particular bladder and liver cancer. Schistosomiasis-infected women are estimated to be three times more likely to contract HIV/AIDS if exposed to the virus. Of the tropical parasitic diseases, schistosomiasis is considered to be the biggest killer after malaria. Some estimates place the toll at more than 170,000 deaths per year, though exact numbers are difficult to track since people often die years after the initial infection from liver or kidney failure or from cancer.

■ ■ ■

In early 1950, soldiers in Communist China's army trained for an invasion of Taiwan (then called Formosa) by swimming in water that turned out to be infested with *S. japonicum*. Between 30,000 and 50,000 men contracted schistosomiasis, delaying the invasion, which was subsequently aborted after the US Seventh Fleet arrived in the Formosa Strait at the start of the Korean War.

The disease was already recognized as part of life in rural China, with an estimated 10 million people infected in Anhui, Fujian, Jiangsu, and Zhejiang Provinces; in parts of Anhui, 80 percent of the inhabitants had schistosomiasis, which also affected a large number of domestic and wild animals. Dr. Yaobi Zhang, an NTD advisor at Helen Keller International who grew up in Anhui Province and started his career working in schistosomiasis control, said the disease was in all twelve provinces in southern China. He recalled seeing pictures of "lots and lots of big belly people"—a sign of advanced schistosomiasis—and "widow villages." Zhang said, "Sometimes in the whole village, you didn't see a man because the men were working in the [rice] fields, and they all got schisto and died."

In the mid-1950s Mao Zedong launched a massive schistosomiasis control program. The only treatments available—basically, poison—were inconsistently effective and sometimes caused dangerous side effects, so the program attempted to break the transmission cycle. Thousands of volunteer students, workers, and peasants collected and killed snails, built dikes, and converted aquatic marshlands into dry fields. "National, provincial, county, the whole system, . . . thousands of staff, just purely working on eliminating schisto," Zhang said. "Surveying, mapping, and then all sorts of methods to kill snails and to treat people. The biggest contribution was the snail control. It was an incredible effort. And it killed the snails and then reduced the transmission."

"China invested so much, so much politically," Zhang said. "Political will: it was unrivaled. Chairman Mao, paramount leader at that time, he said we must eliminate schistosomiasis. There was a huge, huge effort to control. Not only treating people and controlling the snails, there was health education through the schools and the MDA in the domestic animals. It was the whole social effort." China significantly reduced schistosomiasis—but not entirely.

"If you want to kill the snails with chemicals," said Fenwick, who for years tried to reduce schistosomiasis through snail control in Egypt, Sudan, and Tanzania, "you're going to kill fish, you're going to kill other organisms as well. Potentially there are other, nonchemical ways of killing snails—you can introduce ducks which will eat them, you can introduce plants perhaps that are toxic to them, you can introduce fish which may consume them— but none of these control methods have ever eliminated schistosomiasis from any given area." Moreover, the most effective molluscicide (niclosamide) "was a carbon product, and in the 1970s the price of oil rocketed up, and so the cost of the molluscicide also went up."

When construction of the Aswan High Dam was completed in 1970, "the whole surface-water situation in Egypt changed, and so did the number of people infected with schistosomiasis," said Fenwick. "During that same time, there was a huge population explosion in Egypt, and so more and more people were having more and more water contact and, because schistosomiasis is a waterborne disease, intensity and prevalence of infection made it probably the most important disease in Egypt at that time. For example, bladder cancer, which can be caused by schistosomiasis, was the most prevalent cancer in Egypt."

The drug praziquantel entered the market in the late 1970s, a watershed moment akin to the introduction of ivermectin to treat river blindness. "What praziquantel does is strip the tegument—the skin—of the worm, so that suddenly it's exposed," Fenwick said. "The body's defenses then attack the worm." In 1979, Egypt and Israel signed a peace agreement, and "the American government started increasing their aid to Egypt as a sort of political reward. The net result was—having invested in the roads and the telecommunications and the electricity and a few other things—they turned to health. They said, okay, we will put some money into schistosomiasis research and control." Fenwick worked for twelve years with Egypt's Ministry of Health, overseeing research projects and implementing annual nationwide MDAs of praziquantel. "We walked out of there with the knowledge that if the government was willing and interested and motivated, if the drugs were available, and if the financing was available to distribute the drugs, schistosomiasis could be controlled."

Praziquantel is effective and affordable, thanks to Korean pharmaceutical company Shin Poong, which found a way to manufacture it for about ten cents per tablet. From 2007 through 2017 Merck KGaA incrementally increased its donation of praziquantel through WHO from 25 million tablets a year to 250 million tablets annually for school-age children. The trend is moving in the right direction, but distribution still needs to improve. In 2015, of the almost 220 million people in need of this medicine, only 45 percent of children and 14 percent of adults received treatment, according to the *Report of the Tenth Meeting of the WHO Strategic and Technical Advisory Group for Neglected Tropical Diseases*, issued in March 2017. Even supposing that praziquantel could reach everyone who needs it, many people will still engage in activities that reexpose them to infection. While children can be taught not to swim in a particular stream, and people can break the habit of urinating and defecating in or near bodies of water, what about the men and women whose livelihoods require being in that water?

"I depend on Lake Victoria," said Kenyan fisher Boniface Opinya. "Even my wife comes here and fetches water to cook tea for me. We know that it's infected, but we depend on it. If I stop going to the lake, I'll start robbing people all the time. I'll be a thief. Lack of jobs: that's why we are here. I want to be a good character in the village." Before fishing, Opinya had been a teacher for six years, but after not being paid, he had to find other income. "I'm doing my course for driving," he said. "Fishing is what enables me to pay the fee for the course."

I met Opinya in 2013 during a trip with END Fund board members that included helping out at an MDA, learning about the hand-washing and sanitation programs that complement MDAs, visiting labs at KEMRI, and meeting workers at a car wash. Near the town of Kisumu, an unpaved back road led to a small stretch of the eastern shore of Lake Victoria, where several cars and a bus had been driven into the water. Barefoot car washers, carrying buckets and soapy sponges, cleaned the sides of the vehicles, then jumped on top.

One car washer, Simeon Ogola Aquiro, estimated that he spent eight or nine hours in the water every day. "I've worked here for over ten years," he said. "Life is making me continue with it, because I have no other option. Sometimes you may look for another job, but getting that job is not easy."

Both Opinya and Aquiro understood the risks of working in the lake. "Lake Victoria water is not fresh the way it was before," said Opinya. "We don't have things to protect us when we go there. We interact with so many diseases inside there. Bilharzia is the main one. I lost three friends because they didn't know they were suffering from bilharzia."

"The environment we are working in is very dangerous," Aquiro said.

When you are washing vehicles, there are some cuts that you get. There is coldness, especially during rainy season. It forces you to work. My nails, they're cracking. Also the complexion of your skin. Even the hair that people have on their body is turning yellowish. The pores in the body, you find that they are closing. Healthwise, you'll not be normal. When you try to put on anything, like shoes, sand will get between your legs and the shoes, and that will bring damage to your leg. You'll find that the outside skin will be chopped off completely. Barefooted, the way we are, is okay.

The men knew about schistosomiasis—both of them had had it and had been treated with praziquantel administered by KEMRI. "You feel that you are tired," Opinya said. "You have a headache. You have a fever all the time, especially in the evening hours. Sometimes you have diarrhea. An older mother, 60 years plus, people thought she was pregnant, but it was not a pregnancy. It was bilharzia. When the KEMRI came, even me, I was a victim. They took my stool, and they brought my result back. They told me that I am also infected with bilharzia."

"The first day I took the drugs, it's like these things were so many in my stomach," Aquiro said. "After taking the medicine, I was well. I gained more energy. My body became normal. I could continue working. Without treatment, you cannot work here. I would maybe have died. If they find you are infected again, they treat you. Many people will be infected, then reinfected."

■   ■   ■

"What I've learned," said Dr. Mwele Malecela, "is that there's really an importance in being contextual and in really understanding what the issues are." She was talking about Tanzania's LF program, but her words apply to all NTDs. Weak infrastructure, lack of clean water or paved roads, poor sanitation and hygiene, slow economic development, and political instability and conflict all help the diseases thrive. Many people have said that "neglected diseases" should more accurately be termed "diseases of neglected people."

To reduce NTDs, we must address these challenges—a tall order, yet there has been significant, positive change. As head of WHO's Regional Office for Africa, Dr. Moeti has made NTDs an official priority. She came into office in 2016, a few months after APOC's charter had ended; the future was uncertain for the treatment programs that had piggybacked on APOC's Mectizan distribution (e.g., LF treatment). But APOC's replacement, the Expanded Special Project for Elimination of NTDs (ESPEN), now has a formal office in the Regional Office for Africa with its own director, funding, and an action plan to go after the five most prevalent NTDs.

At the national level too, there is progress. Today, most countries with a high burden of NTDs have a national disease control and elimination plan and specific teams within the Ministry of Health that are committed to this work. A standout example is Ethiopia, which in 2013 launched a five-year national plan to tackle the country's eight NTDs.* "Prior to that, neglected tropical

*They are STHs, LF, schistosomiasis, trachoma, river blindness, leishmaniasis, Guinea worm, and podoconiosis.

diseases were not really given attention, and the interventions were not being implemented," said Biruk Kebede Negash, who led the NTD team in Ethiopia's Federal Ministry of Health. A school-based deworming program was scaled up to reach more than 20 million children per year. Hundreds of thousands of people with advanced trachoma have received surgery.

Ethiopia is one of the three most populous countries in Africa, with estimates hovering around 100 million people; more than 75 million of them are thought to be infected with at least one NTD. In 2017, NTDs were incorporated into the curriculum for the frontline community health workers in Ethiopia's Health Development Army, deepening the connection between NTD treatment and the formal health system. As Negash explained, these health workers "understand the cultural views of the community, the cultural perspectives of the community, so they would be very helpful in making sure that the behavioral change interventions are in line with what's on the ground, because what's on the ground is very different from region to region in Ethiopia." Negash is clear about what motivates him: "It's not ethical for humanity to just sit there and watch such burdens affecting the population of the country."

The elimination of schistosomiasis remains a tug-of-war between an "incredibly clever" parasite and people who are dedicated to wiping it out. Despite China's massive snail-control efforts, the disease has resurged there due to population growth and construction in the Yangtze River basin. *S. japonicum* also lives in water buffaloes and cows, so treatment must include veterinary measures.

But in parts of Nigeria, thanks to the work of Dr. Ekwunife and others, schistosomiasis is no longer the "normal" part of life it once was. "When I realized that most of the villagers feel that when they pass blood, it's nothing, they don't care, and it's part of growing up, I took it as a challenge to make sure that it stops," she said.

I planned ahead for admission in the village. I spoke with the headmaster in the schools. Then, on my own, I used my money to purchase medicine, and I treated them. They were reluctant. I took them to the hospital in the city. I scanned their bladder. It wasn't looking like what it was supposed to be. I took photographs of their bladder, and after about six months I scanned their bladder and took the picture of their bladder again, and showed them the picture that showed it was a fine bladder. That was when most of them started to know that actually it was not supposed to be very thin, and they stopped passing blood in urine.

CHAPTER SEVEN

Stone Soup

For thousands of years, practically nothing could be done about neglected tropical diseases. Then, between the 1870s and the 1930s, their parasites and bacteria were identified, and their life cycles and means of transmission were largely uncovered. In the mid-twentieth century, scientists and organizers such as Norman Stoll and Sir John Wilson drew attention to the diseases, but they lacked the ability to institute large-scale treatment and prevention. The late twentieth century saw the advent of drugs that could act against many NTDs, but there remained a global indifference to and ignorance about the prevalence of these diseases. "In the year 2000 hardly a single person was being treated for schistosomiasis in Africa, and it was exactly the same with lymphatic filariasis and trachoma and intestinal worms," said Alan Fenwick. "The exception was river blindness, which had been going with the donated drug. If people had talked of 'neglected diseases' in 1998, they would be talking about malaria and HIV and tuberculosis."

"One is given to wonder, considering that our scientific analysis of the subject is now competent, and the road to control thus clear, whether we are dealing here not with a mercenary, but with a psychological, block against effective action," said Stoll in "This Wormy World," in which he lambasted the inaction of US leaders against trichinosis, a parasitic illness that results from eating undercooked pork. "Perhaps 'trichinosis' is a word of too little odium. Would Americans be equally comfortable in realizing that each 6th among them is harboring garbage worms?" Perhaps the problem was not inertia but branding.

In 2000, world leaders pledged their commitment to the UN's eight Millennium Development Goals (MDGs), which were designed to be a blueprint for action and a mechanism for accountability and coordination. The agreement significantly helped drive progress in many areas, including increased funding and treatment for HIV/AIDS and malaria, reductions in child and maternal mortality, and improved access to primary education. The MDGs asserted that the lives of impoverished people would improve if core issues—health, hunger, education, gender equality, environmental sustainability—were addressed. MDG number six is "combat HIV/AIDS, malaria, and other diseases." But who would notice, who would care, and—significantly—who would fund the research, prevention, and treatment of "other diseases"?

In 2005, a group of scientists who had been working intensively on some of the "other diseases" decided to find a better name. The group included Professor David Molyneux, a parasitologist who had been working on lymphatic filariasis for decades and had served as director of the Liverpool School of Tropical Medicine; Professor Alan Fenwick, one of the world's experts on schistosomiasis and the founder of the Schistosomiasis Control Initiative at Imperial College London; Dr. Lorenzo Savioli, who headed WHO's unit on parasitic diseases and vector control; and Dr. Peter J. Hotez, an American scientist working on vaccines for hookworm and other parasitic diseases (he had also been part of the Rockefeller Foundation's Great Neglected Diseases program and a protégé of Ken Warren). They agreed on "neglected tropical diseases," a nod to the GND program.

Soon after, Molyneux relayed the new name to Dr. Anarfi Asmoah-Baah, who was then WHO's assistant director-general for HIV/AIDS, tuberculosis, and malaria. Asmoah-Baah confirmed the rebranding's success by responding, "I'm going to start a Department of Neglected Tropical Diseases at WHO." Savioli became its inaugural director.

Some argue that the NTD label falls short. "The neglected part, to me, is about the people and not about the diseases," said Don Bundy. It might be more accurate to describe these as diseases of poverty, but many other diseases could fit in that category. Others argue that, thanks to recent increases in funding, these diseases are no longer neglected, but this logic glosses over the fact that significant resources and actions are still needed. Others are puzzled because, technically, not all the diseases are tropical. When I was in Saudi Arabia discussing the high burden of trachoma in Yemen, a local philanthropist asked, "Why is it called a tropical disease? Yemen is not in the tropics." While imperfect, the umbrella term has given advocates and journalists a way to write about, discuss, and reference these diseases.

■   ■   ■

Unless I have a flight to catch, I don't like to get out of bed before dawn, but at 6 a.m. on January 30, 2012, I was at home in Norfolk, Virginia, livestreaming the London Declaration on Neglected Tropical Diseases. Side by side onstage were Bill Gates; the director-general of WHO, Margaret Chan; the CEOs of major pharmaceutical companies Eisai, GlaxoSmithKline, Merck KGaA, MSD, and Sanofi; ministers of health from Mozambique and Tanzania; and officials from the World Bank, DFID, USAID, and the Children's Investment Fund Foundation. The London Declaration was a landmark commitment by these stakeholders, who pledged to dedicate money, resources, and drugs to reach disease-reduction targets recently set by WHO; to work at all levels and across health, education, water, sanitation, and hygiene sectors; and to provide annual progress reports. Never had NTDs reached this high a profile or received this much global attention. The mood in the room, I heard later, was euphoric.

At the time, I was working for Operation Smile, an organization I loved and had served for many years as it grew from a small NGO working in a few countries to a large network with local ownership operating in more than sixty countries, providing surgery and follow-up care to thousands of children with cleft lips and cleft palates. When a recruiter called and encouraged me to apply for the END Fund's CEO position, I hadn't been looking for a job. But I was intrigued by the possibility that I could contribute to helping hundreds of millions of people. I decided to explore the opportunity.

My first interview for the position was scheduled for a few days after the London Declaration, so I was watching the livestream not just out of curiosity but as research. I had been reading every book about NTDs that I could find. My deep dive became a bit of a joke after I was offered the job; I was teased that I was the only candidate who could explain—or even pronounce—the diseases.

Watching the London Declaration announcement was a personal turning point, transforming a tentative interest in joining the END Fund into being completely inspired by the global collaborative approach and the big vision for ending NTDs. At the Harvard School of Public Health, a professor had asked my class, "How can you keep asking, at every step of your work, are you doing the greatest good for the greatest number of people?" I hadn't ever imagined that I might contribute to something that would improve the lives of more than a billion people, but by the end of the livestream, I was hooked.

In London that day, Bill Gates said: "There's a history, a very proud history of involvement [and] donations, and many of the [disease] burdens have come down. But in fact, they haven't come down nearly far enough. What's unique about today is getting everybody on the same page."

Sir Andrew Witty, CEO of GlaxoSmithKline, said: "What you are seeing in the announcement today is a variety of commitments across the board of all of those companies [including] the opening up of compound libraries and intellectual property in partnership with other organizations . . . to really ensure we discover the next generation of potential medicines and treatment for NTDs."

"We are true competitors," said Chris Viehbacher, CEO of Sanofi. "It's not that easy for us to work together commercially. You are talking about research and development, which is where the core secrets of companies are. Sharing libraries of compounds is extraordinarily difficult, and it's only because of the huge need that we've been able to get together. And this is where Bill Gates in particular played such a critical role in catalyzing it."

"This is a special moment for us," said Dr. Alexandre Lourenço Jaime Manguele, minister of health in Mozambique. "That is why we are making a national commitment to fight NTDs by initiating a new integrated program. With planning support from DFID and USAID, we can implement new mass drug administration programs to prevent the spread of these diseases."

"Schistosomiasis is very difficult to pronounce, but it's not impossible to eliminate," said Stefan Oschmann, executive board member (and later CEO) of Merck KGaA. "I'm very happy to be able to officially announce today that we will step up our effort of our drug donation program from 25 million tablets a year to 250 million tablets a year so that WHO will be able to meet their targets. We will also be working on a new pediatric formulation, in particular for preschool-age children, who are particularly vulnerable."

The announcements and endorsements continued. Donors, including the United Arab Emirates, the Lions Club, and Mundo

Sano, came forward with almost US$800 million of new funding commitments for NTD control, including Guinea worm eradication. Eisai increased its donation of DEC to treat LF and river blindness. Bangladesh, Brazil, and Tanzania announced plans to start NTD control programs.

The London Declaration was impressive not only for its spirit of collaboration but for its sheer *logistics*. I'd organized a lot of big events and programs, and I knew how much work and coordination were required. I wondered how the idea had come about and who had done the heavy lifting to pull it off.

∎ ∎ ∎

In 2009, Bill Gates and Dr. Tachi Yamada (the former director of research and development at GlaxoSmithKline, who was heading the Global Health Program at the Gates Foundation) had invited about twenty R&D pharmaceutical companies to come together. At the meeting, they all agreed that they could do more for neglected diseases.

"The question that came to my inbox," said Dr. Julie Jacobson, senior program officer for NTDs at the Gates Foundation, "was, 'So, Julie, what would that look like?' And I'm like, 'We can come up with something—don't you worry!'" MSD's ivermectin donation program was the gold standard—"as much as needed, for as long as needed"—but some of the pharmaceutical companies needed a clearer picture. Jacobson described their response: "Well and good for some of these diseases that are set up for elimination, but what does this mean for others? What does it mean if we give drugs and nobody uses them? We've made commitments before. We need other partners."

She reached out to USAID and DFID. Ministries of Health from recipient countries joined the conversation, as did the World Bank, advocacy and research organizations, and NGOs. In 2012,

WHO released a publication, *Accelerating Work to Overcome the Global Impact of Neglected Tropical Diseases*—nicknamed the "roadmap"—which set targets for the control and elimination of NTDs by 2020.

"We all aligned around the WHO roadmap and said that we would commit to supporting countries in achieving the WHO goals," said Jacobson. "The diseases that became part of the London Declaration were ones where there was a partner willing to put something on the table to make it more likely that we would achieve the WHO's set targets." These included five NTDs manageable by preventive chemotherapy (LF, river blindness, schistosomiasis, intestinal worms, trachoma) and five that required intensive disease management (Chagas disease, Guinea worm, human African trypanosomiasis, leprosy, visceral leishmaniasis).

"There was no broad assessment," Jacobson said. "It's the story of stone soup: 'What are you making?' 'It's stone soup. It's much better with a carrot.' 'I've got a carrot.' 'This is going to be delicious!' 'There isn't enough for everybody, but if we had a potato.' 'I have a potato, and some salt.' Suddenly, there is enough to feed everybody. If anybody thought they had to do this whole thing alone—no way. They're out—especially if you start talking about over a billion people. It isn't possible."

I met Julie Jacobson in April 2012 in Washington, DC, when she was in town to speak at an event called "The Next Frontier in NTD Control" at the National Press Club, just days before I started officially at the END Fund. She warmly welcomed me to the sector and gave me some practical advice—for example, until you learn it all, keep a notecard in your wallet with the diseases' names, vectors, transmission cycles, and drugs used for treatment.

There is hardly anyone who has a clearer, more comprehensive, more inclusive vision of the NTD sector's moving pieces and players than Jacobson. Her commitment to public health, global health, and helping those most neglected is in her blood. Her family's story uniquely embodies the evolution of global health over the past century.

Upon her graduation from medical school in 1994, Jacobson's family gave her a ticket to Karawa, which is "in the northwestern corner of what is now DRC. It was Belgian Congo then; then [it] went to Zaire," she told me. Her grandparents, members of the Swedish Covenant Church, had helped build a hospital there in the 1930s. "My grandfather [Wallace Thornbloom] was a doctor and went to be on the mission field and to start this hospital. My grandmother went to nursing school so that she could join him. They weren't married yet, and there are all these love notes between them: 'Oh, Sarah, I can't wait until I look across the operating theater and you pass me a catgut.'"

Wallace and Sarah were married by a ship's captain three miles off the coast—"because then it's international waters"—and had five children, including Jacobson's mother, Judy, and her uncle Bob Thornbloom, who spearheaded construction of the Zulu Falls hydroelectric plant that powered the hospital and the surrounding area. "Uncle Bob was my hero," Jacobson said. "He was always innovating to make the lives of African women easier."

By the time Julie arrived, nearly sixty years later, the region's potential for prosperity was severely diminished. Deterioration of the political situation had been accompanied by uncontrolled violence and widespread corruption. Despite the surge in AIDS cases, hospitals lacked basic supplies and medicines. "When you wash your hands, there's a big plastic tub of water, because there is no running water," Jacobson recalled. "You have people pour it over your hands, you dry your hands on this towel, and then you take these gloves that have been reused for multiple surgeries.

They dry them out, sterilize them, and powder them so you can get them back on your hand. I remember pulling a glove on and hearing a pop—and silence. It was that one last glove, and they didn't know when they were going to get more."

Jacobson worked under Dr. Roger Thorpe, who had been trained by her grandfather. "[Thorpe] fell into a huge depression while I was there," she said. "It was the first time that he had realized how bad it was and how things had slipped so far backwards. I would ask a simple question and the profundity of that question—'When is the chemo going to arrive?'—was overwhelming for him." She saw that the work done by her grandfather and uncle—"all those years and lives dedicated to this"—was unraveling. "It was still a Band-Aid."

One patient with an enormous hydrocele that had been caused by LF walked for *three months* to reach the hospital for a hydrocelectomy, which Jacobson helped perform. This kind of case and that moment when the last glove tore on her hand made her realize she was at "the wrong end of the spectrum of fighting the disease. By the time we're getting people into the hospital, we're already at the losing end of the battle. What we need to do is move much further up and understand the prevention piece. Unless we can prevent these things, we're never going to be able to help people. The quality of their lives has already been demolished by infectious diseases that are easily preventable and should not be an issue."

One afternoon, she heard airplanes. "Airplanes never came over. I was outside and people were running around and talking and kids were playing soccer, and everybody stopped and just looked up, and everybody knew that something was not good. This was when the Rwandan refugee crisis was happening—and all the massacres."

With her uncle, Jacobson flew to Nairobi to volunteer. She was sent to Goma, which is on the DRC side of the border with Rwanda.

Here I am, three months out of medical school, and I'm put in charge of a camp of 200,000 people with a cholera epidemic. There's no water, and all we did every day was count bodies and try to figure out what to do with them because you can't even bury because you're on lava. We just arranged for people to take the dead bodies and pile them on the other side of the road—you can't imagine the smell—and then try and create order. I elected somebody who made eye contact with me and spoke English. I would say, "Okay, you're now my chief, and I need you to help me organize this." I got a couple of people to stand as guard so we had space, because as soon as you came, it was just everybody around you—it was total panic—and create a barrier with a piece of string that people couldn't cross so that we could bring our supplies out.

We had antibiotics, and all night long I would pack up little packs of antibiotics. If people could sit up, it was oral rehydration salts, spoonful by spoonful, with a family member giving them that to keep them alive. And taking people that could walk—there was a Médecins Sans Frontières tent that was four kilometers down the road—somebody had to get them to the MSF tent. If they couldn't stand up, those were the people that I cared for. That's the way I triaged: "Can you stand? Okay, then you have to make it to the tent." Then it was just going around giving IV fluids. I was seeing 150 people a day. Then we learned the outbreak of cholera that ripped through the camp was drug-resistant, so the antibiotics were useless.

"I was fortunate to have seen," she said. "Once you've seen, you can't go back. You can't pretend."

After ten months abroad, she returned to the States ("It was Christmas time. It was complete over-the-top everything: sugar and gifts and people caring about ridiculous things") to complete her medical residency in family practice ("I wanted to be able to do everything: an appendectomy, deliver a baby, and take care of somebody at the end of life"). This was followed by the CDC's Epidemic Intelligence Service program, with a focus on disaster response ("Listening to the radio and something just happened in the Dominican Republic, and I would say, 'I'm glad I already have my bag packed'").

While at the international global health nonprofit PATH from 2000 to 2007, Jacobson worked to implement a vaccination program for Japanese encephalitis (JE) in India. She recalled "going to hospitals and seeing two kids to a bed, seizing in a pool of urine, and unconscious." It happens every year, local doctors told her. The rainy season brings an increase in mosquitoes carrying the JE virus. "But there's a vaccine!" she responded. In fact, there was a new and improved single-dose vaccine out of China, giving lifetime protection. "The manufacturer we were working with in China agreed to honor our public-sector price before we had signed any paperwork because I said, 'If you tell them you are willing to honor this price now, I know we can make this happen in India.'" Eight months after India's commitment, the vaccine was introduced, and 9.3 million people were immunized. The resulting data convinced the Indian Parliament to make the immunization routine. According to Jacobson, as of 2016, 120 million people in Asia have received the vaccine.

In 2007, Jacobson joined the Gates Foundation. "I thought that experience, of getting [the JE vaccine] out there, was really important for the foundation to understand. There was so much focus on products. Getting them out there was where it was really hard and complicated." Given the choice of which program to join, she chose neglected diseases. "In all the things that I have done, I have always worked with the neglected areas or the neglected people," she said. "That has always been my piece."

■ ■ ■

The idea to create a foundation dates from 1993, when Bill and Melinda Gates went on safari in Kenya's Maasai Mara National Reserve. They saw plenty of wild animals, but the indelible impression was of the disease and poverty that permeated rural African life. "I remember peering out a car window at a long line of women walking down the road with big jerricans of water on their heads," Bill later wrote in an essay for *Wired* magazine. "How far away do these women live? we wondered. Who's watching their children while they're away?" In an interview with *Scientific American*, he elaborated: "That trip got me thinking about how much nutrition people there have, how people live—sometimes not even being able to afford shoes—why so many children die and the different tiers of social development."

People in the Gateses' situation—Westerners on vacation shocked at the poverty in a foreign land—often give to the village they visited, for example, by supporting a local, community-based NGO focusing on health or education. Being the founder of Microsoft, a man who often thinks in terms of data and on a big scale, Bill Gates went home determined to make a contribution, but rather than donate to an individual person or place, he and Melinda looked at the system. How could their vast fortune and unique access to technology be used to improve *many* lives? How could they change the big picture? Gates was profoundly affected by *Investing in Health*, the World Bank's 1993 *World Development Report*, which stated plainly that 12 million children died every year due to entirely preventable diseases such as pneumonia, diarrhea, and malaria. "That was the first time it dawned on me," Gates wrote in *Wired*, "that it's not hundreds of different diseases causing most of the problem—it's a pretty finite number. And I was surprised by the huge disparity between poor countries, where 20 percent of children were dying before the age of five, and rich countries where that number is more like half a percent."

Several Gates family foundations were established in the 1990s—the William H. Gates Foundation, the Gates Library Foundation, and the Gates Learning Foundation—and in 2000 they were rolled into one entity, the Bill & Melinda Gates Foundation. In 2006, Warren Buffett pledged much of his fortune to the foundation, almost doubling its granting capacity. Its current endowment is approximately $40 billion, and its stated priorities are global health and poverty and US education.

"The largest program [in the early days] was the library program," said Dr. David Brandling-Bennett, formerly a senior program officer who worked first on tropical diseases and then on malaria. "Global health was around forty people. Infectious diseases was about ten people. And there was nutrition and child survival; they were fairly small."

"They would hire young tech guys to fly to libraries around the country and plug in the internet," recalled Gabrielle Fitzgerald, who worked on program advocacy at the foundation from 2004 to 2014. "It was one of the foundation's early lessons, that you can't actually do that because then you're not building capacity, and then when it breaks, you have no solution."

From the start, the Gates Foundation supported work on diseases that later would be labeled "neglected tropical diseases": schistosomiasis, LF, intestinal worms, leishmaniasis, and human African trypanosomiasis. The department—first called Neglected and Other Diseases, then Neglected Infectious Diseases—didn't have a formal strategy of development. "Only in the coming years did they get organized into what were called strategic program teams," said Fitzgerald.

"These seemed like classical diseases that required some sort of attention on the part of the foundation," Brandling-Bennett said.

It was often a point of debate as to why the foundation supported work on the diseases and whether the foundation should do so. I think the principal reason was that these were diseases of the poorest; they had some role in perpetuating poverty and the disadvantages that people had. Even if they were not suffering something frank, like disabling elephantiasis, the effect of these diseases on populations was significant. But the overall burden was not as high as, say, for malaria or diarrheal diseases or pneumonia. Also, then, what should one do with these diseases? The foundation, I think correctly, was not in the business of just funding programs to control and reduce these diseases. At that time, elimination was not something we talked about for pretty much any disease, except perhaps polio.

Initially the infectious diseases team was six people, who would sit around a table and read letters of inquiry. Brandling-Bennett recalled:

Occasionally, some nice great idea would come up and we'd say, "That may be worth exploring." But a lot of it was thinking about what was going to make a difference to an approach. And who would we consider would be a group that could undertake this work? We'd often be in discussions with the CDC or The Carter Center or WHO and be saying, "This is what we think might be worth doing. What do you think?" We'd go back and forth about an idea. They might initially approach us with an idea. Often it was, "We need funding for this." And we'd say, "We don't just fund things. What are we going to learn that will lead to more effective approaches and actually get the job done that you want to do, rather than just do good things because you should do them?"—which was fine, but not really what the foundation was about. The foundation has been justifiably quite clear that investments it wants to make are ones that are game changing.

In the early days, NTDs registered as a relatively low priority, but given how little worldwide funding was going to these diseases at the time, the Gates Foundation had an outsize influence. More organizations and government funding agencies followed suit, eventually bringing more resources and greater attention. "There are so few investors [in NTDs] that the Gates Foundation could really be a huge driver in it, more so than HIV, where we were a small fish in a big pond. We could be this huge fish in this small pond," Fitzgerald said. The downside, Brandling-Bennett said, was the pervasive idea that "if the foundation's not doing it, then it's not important. In some ways, others should be investing in something *because* the foundation is not." To incentivize other philanthropists, the Gates Foundation often gives support by matching or leveraged funds.

"The goal in much of what we do," Gates wrote in *Wired*, "is to provide seed funding for various ideas. Some will fail. We fill a function that government cannot—making a lot of risky bets with the expectation that at least a few of them will succeed. At that point, governments and other backers can help scale up the successful ones, a much more comfortable role for them."

There have been failures, including a vaccine for visceral leishmaniasis, in which the foundation invested tens of millions of dollars. But there have been far more successes. The foundation played a pivotal role in the Global Alliance for Vaccines and Immunizations, which has helped increase vaccine coverage globally and significantly reduced child mortality. It has been a leader in the fight to eradicate polio, combat malaria, and develop new tools, diagnostics, and drugs for a whole range of diseases that plague the developing world.

In the early 2000s, various NGOs were trying to scale up the delivery of donated NTD drugs, but the different programs were often treating the same people—and sometimes using the same drug. Albendazole was used for intestinal worms, LF, and river blindness; many people with schistosomiasis also had LF or river blindness; almost everyone with an NTD had intestinal worms—but each disease had its own program with its own staff, data, and treatment programs.

"Why are we funding separate programs?" asked the foundation's twenty-fourth hire, Dr. Regina Rabinovich, director of the infectious diseases unit. "Can you actually integrate these programs?" The idea had been floated before, at The Carter Center and elsewhere, but nobody had undertaken the effort at scale.

"I issued a call for proposals," Brandling-Bennett said, "for ideas about how one could actually develop and test integrated programs. This gradually got traction, and it's fair to say that now an integrated approach is a normal approach for these, with varying degrees of success. It does require that people understand the value of working together on these diseases. The programs were often separate and sometimes they were in separate departments: if there was a vector involved, then it might be in the vector control department, whereas in other diseases it would be under somebody else's control."

"It's about time," Mwele Malecela recalled the district workers saying in response to Tanzania's integration of its LF program with intestinal worms, schistosomiasis, and river blindness. "We were wondering, 'What's wrong with you people?' You would come with the LF program, another person would come with the oncho program, and this would be weeks apart. We thought it was a donor requirement that you can't combine the programs."

■ ■ ■

"The foundation is built on the premise that all lives have equal value, that every person deserves the chance to live a healthy and productive life, and we fund according to that mission," said Dr. Katey Owen, director of the foundation's Neglected Tropical Diseases Division. "The other spaces where pharma is not going to step in and create solutions or where there's not a clear market, where there's been a market failure—those are spaces where the Gates Foundation has more interest, in general, in stepping in. And of course, those spaces where there is a very high burden of disease, both morbidity and mortality." Referring to disability-adjusted life years (DALYs)—a measurement that reflects the impact of both early mortality and ongoing morbidity—Owen remembered "the number of times that I've been in meetings with Bill where he has said, 'We're dollars-per-DALY people.' Almost every single meeting I'm in with him, that's what he says." In other words, the foundation's goal of making the maximum impact on improving health is ever present.

In 2017, the NTD team arranged a series of education sessions with Gates. "We talked about 'this is what an NTD program is,'" Owen recalled. "This is how we're thinking strategically about spending our dollars on NTDs. This is what a mass drug administration looks like, from the training to the advocacy to the actual delivery of the drugs, to the measurement and evaluation."

At one session, Dr. Nana-Kwadwo Biritwum, who was then the NTD program manager for Ghana (he has since joined the Gates Foundation), brought a dose pole, a measuring stick used to assess the number of pills a person should take based on their height. He approached Bill Gates and said, "Can I please ask you to stand up?

I'm going to share with you how this would happen if we were visiting any house in Tanzania or any place in Ghana." Gates stood up and was measured on the dose pole. Then, based on his height, Biritwum handed Gates several tablets of praziquantel and said, "Okay, we expect you to take that drug."

Owen recalled, "Bill's response was, Whoa—those drugs are big. That's a lot of drugs. He immediately started asking questions. Why are they formulated this way? How come there's not a single drug? We started asking questions about social mobilization: you come to someone's house without any education whatsoever, and you put a drug in their hand and you expect them to take it?"

A few months later, Gates traveled to Tanzania to see what an MDA looked like on the ground. He accompanied community health workers going house to house. Owen recalled:

> He asked questions along the way. Things like: Oh, you have electrical wires. How much electricity do you have in this village? What's the consistency of that? Noticing things about the water sanitation and hygiene—so you have latrines in the certain areas. How do you position these, in terms of the community? It was maybe six or seven houses, and we ended in the pharmacy. In the pharmacy they had all of the records. Bill is very keen on data—data recording and also quality management of the program. He asked more questions. So, you record every name. Do you ever go back and track whether or not it's the exact same name from one administration to the next? (The answer to that was no.) How do you know how many names you actually should have versus how many names you do have? (The answer to that was, we know the community.) What about when you don't know the community? (The answer was, we always know the community.) He asked questions about remote areas. There was a remote settlement up in the hills, and he asked, so who goes and sees those people? Are

those people missed, or are they actually not missed, and how do you know?

Describing the experience in a November 6, 2017, post on his *Gates Notes* blog, Bill Gates wrote:

> Walking from door to door in the village with the health workers, I was struck that perhaps the most important element of the program is trust. Taking the medicine is strictly voluntary, making it important that the health workers distributing it earn the confidence of the community. The health workers I met certainly had. They were knowledgeable, passionate about their work, and clearly cared about the community they were serving. At each home, they took the time to explain the goal of the program and address any of the villagers' questions or concerns. Thanks to their hard work the latest survey of lymphatic filariasis in their district showed that the cycle of transmission had been broken. For the first time, the village was not at risk of the disease.

■ ■ ■

The fifth anniversary of the London Declaration was held in April 2017 at WHO headquarters in Geneva. The gathering had mushroomed from a few hundred in 2012 to almost 800. Several significant benchmarks were celebrated: the number of people treated annually (for at least one NTD) had grown from around 727 million to just over 1 billion. The number of people at risk and needing treatment had dropped by 300 million. More than 150 world leaders had signed up for the UN Sustainable Development Goals, which included NTD elimination by 2030 as a global priority.

A month later, Dr. Margaret Chan stepped down as WHO's director-general after many years of championing and supporting NTD control and elimination efforts. In her final address to the World Health Assembly, she highlighted NTDs:

The relevance of WHO was most dramatically demonstrated during last month's global partners meeting on the neglected tropical diseases. . . .This is one of the most effective partnerships, also with industry, in the modern history of public health. The fact that, in 2015, nearly one billion people received free treatments that protect them from diseases that blind, maim, deform, and debilitate has little impact on the world's geopolitical situation. The people being protected are among the poorest in the world. But judging from the massive amounts of media coverage, which included entry into the Guinness World Records for the most medication donated, this was a success story that the world was hungry to hear.

CHAPTER EIGHT

Unfrozen Moment

"Gates Finds Controversy Even in Works of Charity" ran the headline of a June 12, 2006, *Financial Times* article by Andrew Jack. Noting recent criticisms of the Bill & Melinda Gates Foundation—not enough transparency in grant decisions, a shift from "saving lives now" to development of drugs and technology—the article cited Professor Alan Fenwick as "among those who stress that many of the world's most neglected diseases, such as lymphatic filariasis and schistosomiasis, two parasitic ailments, do not need innovation but simply modest funding and a little imagination in order to distribute drugs to those in need."

Among those reading the article that morning were Christopher Chandler and Alan McCormick, financial investors from Legatum, a private investment firm based in Dubai. Intrigued, McCormick called Imperial College London and was put through to Fenwick. A mere fifty cents per person was the annual cost of preventing diseases such as intestinal worms and schistosomiasis, Fenwick explained. The bulk of the cost was delivery, and by combining drug distributions to treat different parasites simultaneously, the per-treatment cost could be even lower.

Legatum was created from the amicable demerger of Sovereign Global, which had been founded in 1986 by two New Zealanders in their early 20s: brothers Christopher and Richard Chandler. Sovereign started out in Hong Kong real estate in 1987. Most investors didn't see the point of putting money into the territory, which was about to be returned from Britain to China. With profit from the sale of their family's chain of New Zealand department stores, the Chandlers bought and renovated buildings in Hong Kong's central business district. When they sold their properties four years later, their net worth was more than $40 million. They spent the next decades "looking for opportunities and markets that had been overlooked or were misunderstood or people were afraid of," Christopher Chandler said.

Sovereign was not afraid of volatility. In 1991, when Brazil opened to foreign investment for the first time, the company bought millions of shares in telephone and electricity companies, staying put even after stocks plunged as President Fernando Collor de Mello was impeached for a kickback scheme. Sovereign left Brazil in 1993 with a fivefold return on its investment.

Following the collapse of the Soviet Union, Sovereign not only invested in Russian companies, it took on two governance battles —first at the country's biggest steelmaker, Novolipetsk Metallurgical Kombinat, and then at Gazprom, the top gas producer in the world, accusing board members of selling products at below-market prices to third-party export agents owned by company managers. Despite intimidation efforts and the 1998 collapse of the ruble, Sovereign Global stayed and won both fights.

Sovereign went into countries that were uncharted investment territory, where there was little or no history of objective analysis or corporate accountability; it performed its own analyses, created its own metrics, and, once the decision to invest had been made, bet big. Its stake in Russia totaled $194 million, making Sovereign the holder of the largest foreign portfolio in the country at the time. In the early 2000s, the company put more than $1 billion into Japan. "Narrow and deep" was the approach: no more than ten equity positions at one time. Diversification, according to Chandler, was "deworsification." "Our specialty," he said, "was moving in to invest in markets at times of transition, because during periods of transition, everything becomes possible. Transitions are unfrozen moments. Before everything refreezes, you can get involved and see what's possible."

NTDs are in an unfrozen moment. Globally, they affect more than a billion people. Within a village, they can debilitate a majority of the population, preventing children from attending school and adults from working, causing lasting repercussions for the local community and nationally. This unfrozen moment is an unprecedented chance for NTDs to be brought under control as the result of advancements in technology, donations of effective medicines, growing awareness, collaboration across sectors, and increased funding. But more is needed: ideas, people, innovation, funding. Never has there been a better time to "get involved and see what's possible."

■ ■ ■

Legatum's strategy of looking for unfrozen moments has applied to not only financial but philanthropic investments in sectors where the firm's contribution could have high leverage, where its involvement would be money but also ideas. Sovereign Global, and subsequently Legatum, regularly donated a portion of its fortune to charity with support from Geneva Global, a philanthropic advisory organization that was established by Sovereign. Geneva Global has a "very crude metric," McCormick said, "which we call 'cost per life-change.'"

> We try to look at the direct beneficiaries that we impact through our philanthropy and then divide it by the amount of money that we spend, and it gives us a cost per life-change result. The average cost of our life-changes was between $12 and $14, so it piqued our imagination when we heard that for fifty cents you could change

a life [affected by NTDs]. When we started to dig into it and see, actually, the depth of the change that you could bring to some of these
lives, it was quite profound. . . . The way that we view the world is
ROI, return on investment. We feel like we're stewards of capital.
You can invest it and get a financial return, or you can give it and get a
psychosocial return. In category 1, you recycle the money. Category
2—the money is gone, but we take great delight in figuring out, if we
have a dollar to spend, what is the optimal way to spend that dollar?

When Geneva Global expanded into offering philanthropic
advice to organizations other than Sovereign, Chandler was surprised to see that other philanthropists cared little beyond cutting
the check. "Over 90 percent of the people were honest enough to say,
'Actually we don't really feel that the outcomes are that important. It's
much more the act of giving that's important.'" The rigor and stan-
dards usually brought to their profession seemed not to apply to
philanthropy. "That never rang true with us. We always felt that
the responsibility wasn't to invest; it was to invest wisely."

Fenwick and McCormick met in person in the same Imperial
College building where Alexander Fleming had discovered penicillin in 1928. With a $30 million grant from the Gates Foundation,
Fenwick had founded SCI in 2002. After working for five years
in six African countries, SCI had demonstrated that schistosomiasis could be controlled using praziquantel through mass drug
administration. Now, SCI and other NGOs were advocating to
integrate the treatment of schistosomiasis, LF, river blindness,
trachoma, and intestinal worms. Their hope was to dramatically
drive down the cost per treatment. The Gates Foundation had not
renewed SCI's grant, at that time choosing to move away from
funding direct MDA, which was becoming USAID's focus. Without that money, SCI was concerned that its work would stall.

"I was struck by several things," McCormick said. "First, the heavy lifting on these diseases had already been done. The diseases had been mapped in a number of countries. The drugs existed and were ready for distribution. Second was the opportunity to try the new integrated MDA approach. Third, we could potentially catalyze a movement focusing on these forgotten diseases and, ultimately, forgotten people. Rarely can a philanthropic investment be so catalytic and accomplish so many things in one go."

How could Legatum get involved? The majority of untreated NTDs were in Africa. Could the firm fund a project integrating treatment in some of the smaller countries, like Burundi and Rwanda? "We saw the opportunity to create a case study on these two," McCormick said, "and if we could prove the case study, that would be an opportunity to bring other investors in."

"I was a little bit skeptical," Fenwick later said of the meeting. "But I was going to Africa the following week, so when they expressed an interest in Rwanda and Burundi, I was able to talk to the ministers of health."

True to form, Legatum went big, allocating an $8.9 million grant to Geneva Global to support a coalition of partners to deliver an integrated NTD treatment program over three years in the two countries. In Rwanda, more than 65 percent of all children had intestinal worms; in districts near lakes, schistosomiasis was inescapable. Many households and schools lacked functional latrines and a nearby source of clean water. Both countries moved quickly, scaling up from mapping and administering limited, pilot MDAs in year 1 to 90 percent coverage of at-risk populations by year 3. More than 8.5 million people were treated (with a focus on preschool and school-age children and on women of child-bearing age who were not in the first trimester of a pregnancy) at an average cost of twenty cents per person. Thousands of doctors, lab technicians, community health workers, and teachers were trained. Comic strips and radio shows disseminated information.

"The child that did not take the medicine, you can see they are not physically well," said Jmu Mbonyiintwari, headmaster of the Rwesero School near Muhazi Lake in Rwanda. "Their belly is protruding and popping out. We can see the child isn't following well what the teacher says. You find the child will often get sick. . . . They are in pain instead of studying. The child who has taken the medicine pays more attention in class. You can see the child is growing. You can see it in their faces. They are better." The prevalence of schistosomiasis at the Rwesero School was 69.5 percent in 2008. In 2014, it was zero.

■ ■ ■

In the mid-2000s, NTDs started to gain more recognition. Under President George W. Bush, the United States stepped up its global health funding, notably through the President's Emergency Plan for AIDS Relief (PEPFAR) in 2003 and the President's Malaria Initiative in 2005. In 2006, NTDs came on the Bush administration's radar. The fact that some of these diseases could be eliminated was appealing. Former president Jimmy Carter and The Carter Center had been working on Guinea worm since 1986 and had reduced the disease's prevalence so dramatically each year that eradication was a real possibility.

Peter Hotez and his colleagues at the newly formed Global Network for NTDs dove into advocacy. Receptive US audiences included Tommy Thompson, former secretary of Health and Human Services; Senator Sam Brownback; Senator Patrick Leahy and his longtime aide Tim Rieser; Anthony Fauci, head of the National Institute of Allergy and Infectious Diseases; and Mark Dybul, who led the implementation of PEPFAR. David Molyneux and Fenwick did the same in London with members of Parliament and at the Department for International Development (DFID), which increased funding commitments for trachoma, LF, and schistosomiasis. In 2006, for the first time, Congress included NTDs in the global health budget. They were allotted $15 million, enough for USAID to start an NTD program.

In 2009 that funding increased to $25 million. It was $65 million in 2010. Despite this investment and critical funding during this time from the Gates Foundation, gaps remained. At a 2010 NTD stakeholders' meeting at the White House, McCormick felt there was still room for greater efficiency and innovation—two specialties of the private sector.

The four Legatum partners (Chandler, McCormick, Mark Stoleson, and Philip Vassiliou) and Doug Balfour, CEO of the recently independent Geneva Global, decided to create a private philanthropic fund for NTDs. Their vision was to pool capital from individual, foundation, and corporate donors, relying on specialized technical knowledge and on fund managers who would track NTD partners and opportunities. The fund would make high-leverage, high-impact investments. Instead of backing one organization and helping it scale, the fund would take a systems view and try to boost an entire sector. In the same way that a fund manager gives an investor access to an asset class, the newly minted END Fund would give donors knowledge about NTDs and NTD organizations, saving the donors the work of doing the due diligence and sector research themselves. A new model of philanthropy was envisioned: many entrepreneurs have a liquidity event on the sale of their business and then create foundations and hire staff to evaluate grants; the END Fund could play that outsourced role. It would use tools of the investment industry to drive accountability and stay nimble, flexible, and focused on impact. Geneva Global hosted, nurtured, and eventually spun off the END Fund into a separate organization.

William I. Campbell, a senior advisor at J. P. Morgan, came on board as the END Fund's chair. Campbell had met the Legatum team in Rwanda in 2009, when they were checking on the progress of Legatum's investment. After several years of exploring various projects in Africa, Campbell was looking for a way to support scaling low-cost, transformational interventions that would improve people's lives. By chance, he met some of the Legatum team at a bar in Kigali's Serena Hotel, and they quickly discovered a shared vision for business and philanthropy. Campbell brought funds, connections, and—perhaps most valuable—the hard-won perspective of a philanthropist wanting to do more than write a check, who had encountered altruism's real-world complexities. For years, he had kept in his office the architectural plans for a failed fistula hospital in Niger, into which the Campbell Family Foundation had invested significant time and funds—as a reminder of how hard it is to get philanthropy right.

■ ■ ■

"The Long Road to Elimination of Neglected Tropical Diseases" ran the headline of an April 18, 2017, *Financial Times* article by Andrew Jack—the same journalist and publication that had caught the attention of Alan McCormick eleven years prior. Among those who saw the article, part of a special report on NTDs, was Tope Lawani, who was on a flight home to London from Marseille. Lawani grew up in Oyo State, Nigeria, attended college and graduate school in the United States, and in 2004 cofounded Helios Investment Partners, a multibillion-dollar private equity firm that invests exclusively in Africa. Lawani recalled his response to the article:

> I was born and raised in Nigeria, and I went to secondary school there. Among the topics that you learn is biology, and you learn about all of these tropical diseases. So they were actually quite familiar, at least from a schoolboy's standpoint; growing up in the nicer parts of town, you weren't inundated every day with the

practical realities of the existence of these diseases. Fast-forward thirty-three years on, and I realized that these things are almost as prevalent as they were then. In an age where so much progress had been made on problems that seemed to be a lot more intractable, like HIV and even malaria—that these diseases would still exist and still be taking lives or dramatically reducing the quality of life in so many places—I was pretty astounded by that.

After seeing the END Fund referenced in the *Financial Times* article, Lawani reached out directly to me. Initially I wondered if he had mistaken the END Fund for a financial fund, but I came to realize that he was attracted to the fund model of tackling neglected tropical diseases. Lawani liked the idea of supporting a whole portfolio of investments and organizations across the sector, each with a tailored approach to the local problem:

Execution is the hardest thing in Africa: actually getting stuff done. There's no shortage of good ideas; there's no shortage of anything. It's just execution. Can you actually do it? The way we think about our business—when you're investing with a relatively lean team across a continent of fifty-four countries with a fairly large portfolio of companies, I think all the time about how do you project yourself, or sort of force-multiply in a way that enables you to keep maximum control and visibility on the things that you're doing, while doing more at the same time. It's all about operations.

The END Fund could have said, "We'll raise some money, and we'll have a team that is present in a number of countries, and we'll try to do the thing that we do." And that would be mightily challenging because you'd have to become expert in Nigeria, expert in Zimbabwe, expert in Ghana, expert in all of these places that have completely disparate needs and realities. You'd have to—in that example—yourself go find someone as an employee who would be knowledgeable about Zimbabwe, passionate about Zimbabwe, entrepreneurial enough to do all of the things you're trying to do, and I can tell you that you would not succeed in doing that yourself.

The model that the END Fund has chosen is: find the entrepreneurial, passionate person in Zimbabwe, who gets the local reality and who has execution capability (albeit on a localized level)—they're not the same person who will do it for you in Uganda, but they don't need to be. Have those people on the ground doing their thing and bringing the passion that they bring and then have you essentially be in the business of giving ammunition and firepower and structure to these organizations. The model that the END Fund is deploying is leveraged in the sense of being able to do increasingly more with disproportionately less.

The focus of Helios's business also motivated Lawani's instant desire to get involved:

We're African specialists. We're very much committed to the continent. We're not short-termists, and therefore we're generally supportive of the greater good in the markets in which we operate. There are a number of sectors in which we invest; we do a lot, for example, in financial services. We've historically been the largest shareholder in a bank in East Africa called Equity Bank. Equity Bank is unusual in the sense that its principal focus is on the so-called bottom of the pyramid. From Equity Bank's perspective, not only does it have a large customer base—I believe more than 10 million depositors, or customers, across Kenya, DRC, Rwanda, Tanzania, and South Sudan—but that population is certainly more at risk because of living conditions and the quality of public health in the region. It's in Equity Bank's interest, for its own good, to make sure that its population is healthy and productive and going to work and making money. And therefore they can deposit more money in the bank and borrow more money from the bank, and the bank makes more money.

Another example of Helios's investments is Fertilizers and Inputs Holding B.V., a company that distributes fertilizer, crop protections, and seeds. "It serves tens of thousands of farmers and cooperatives in about eight countries in Africa," Lawani said. "Your actual end customer is the small-holder farmer who's living in an environment and working in a profession, at least in the African context, where there is some susceptibility to some of these neglected tropical diseases. In the most direct sense, you need farmers in the fields, working and being productive, if you're going to make money." Put another way: "If your customers are sick and dying, you're not going to make a lot of money."

■ ■ ■

In 2007 USAID chose Mali—along with Burkina Faso, Ghana, Niger, and Uganda—to pilot the integrated treatment of NTDs. Prior to the 2012 coup d'état, Mali's NTD program was a shining example of what was possible. Coverage was up. Costs were down. Prevalence was down. The program could be replicated. In the aftermath of the coup, the END Fund's private, unrestricted funds provided unique flexibility and independence.

"For USAID, it was one of those moments where it changed the perception around the END Fund and the role of private philanthropy and how quick and agile it can be," said Emily Wainwright, who headed USAID's NTD program. "Obviously, the US government is not agile and has political considerations. It was kind of a pleasant surprise. We wanted Mali to win. We didn't want people to suffer just because of the political environment. It was a great opportunity to see in real time how it all dovetailed together nicely." Wainwright had seen private philanthropy not work:

It can be just big hearts wanting to get involved in something but not taking the context into account. I've seen private philanthropy give money or resources and not understand what's happening on the ground, not looking at how these investments support the Ministry of Health, or what's going on in the larger context. There can be duplications of effort and double-paying for things, when that's not what we really need. And then it can distract people; it can derail well-developed agendas and progress, depending on the magnitude of the resources.

Actually, some giving can put a huge amount of strain on the governments and people in communities to figure out how to manage the resources. There are all sorts of unintended consequences. In Indonesia after the tsunami, people were donating all these clothes, and what it wound up doing in the microfinance field was all the people who were tailors and made clothes, it totally ruined their livelihoods, because there were all these free clothes in the country.

Wainwright's remarks reminded me of hearing Ellen Johnson Sirleaf, who was president of Liberia at the time, describe her government's philanthropy coordination office. If philanthropists want to come in, they should first meet with that office, which can give some guidance and connect potential donors to the right government ministries to partner and coordinate with. She offered the example of people coming in and wanting to set up a school. Liberia needs schools—but the country has an education plan, which includes where to put new schools. If philanthropists work in alliance with the government and build a school in a place that needs one, then the government will pay the teachers and put electricity there.

USAID supports governments as they start and continue NTD programs. "Never underestimate how important and how time-consuming donor coordination and program implementation is," Wainwright said, "but it needs to be done." Down the line, USAID helps countries determine if they are succeeding. "One of the great misconceptions is that USAID only supports MDA. If we've supported your MDA, we're going to help you evaluate whether you've eliminated the disease, and we'll definitely help you put your dossier together. What's the point of going to all that effort and not confirming it? Not finishing the agenda doesn't make any sense to me."

The END Fund's participation in Mali, Wainwright said, "had been a real selling point for us inside USAID, to be able to show an example of how private philanthropy can work. I've had the experience of seeing private philanthropy be something that can raise money. It can and should be able to add value. But it sometimes gets very disconnected from what's going on and winds up being kind of a distraction. Or, quite frankly, it can be in some cases even destabilizing, and I think Mali was an excellent example of how that was not true, not true at all."

The NTD sector is small enough that each participant makes a great impact. The END Fund's role is different from that of The Carter Center or SCI or Sightsavers, and all of those differ greatly from USAID or DFID. "There's nothing worse than saying you're the only ones in the space," said Wainwright. The NTD donor base is "not your typical cast of characters. It makes people think twice: Wow, there's clearly something here. Something is capturing people's imagination in a way we hadn't originally considered." Part of the vision of the END Fund is to help capture people's imagination about ending a problem, and then provide an easy on-ramp for them to get involved, whether engaging new donors, small or large, or helping new program partners join the efforts. I remember thinking early in my NTD days that as a community we should always have the humility to think that the smartest person might not have entered the room yet, that the right set of skills and the perspective to really reach the end may not yet be part of the global efforts.

Wainwright started at USAID in 1997 and worked in many areas, including child survival, micronutrients, tuberculosis, and environmental health. She joined the NTD team in 2011 because she could see that "this was working. Something amazing was going to happen." Moreover, "most everything that we focus on in the health sector [at USAID] is about reducing mortality, and this was an opportunity to actually work on a program that improves quality of life."

From the start, the NTD team at USAID was mandated to be small: about five people in Washington, DC, and no staff at the country level. At the time, "there was a fatigue around these really big funds and huge programs that got very bureaucratic." While the staff is lean, the impact is huge. "I like scale," Wainwright said. "I don't like pilot projects, and I don't like, in the field of public health, thinking small. My favorite thing about this program is it is big. We are not helping 50,000 people; we are not helping 150,000 people. In a given year, [USAID-supported programs] are reaching out and impacting the lives of over 150 million people a year. I've worked in a village, and I like that, but I don't want it to be just the village. I want it to be everybody."

■　■　■

When I see the manifestations of NTDs, I feel sad that anyone should have to carry those burdens, I feel shocked because the diseases are terrible, and I'm angry at the neglect. When I study the diseases' transmission cycles, however, I am amazed. The parasites and bacteria behind NTDs have incredibly intricate, often ingenious, life cycles. They change shape. They hide from the human immune system. They can remain undetected for years.

They have survived while many other species have gone extinct. These microscopic creatures pose a giant, complex challenge. Outsmarting them depends on our best medicine, technology, and collaboration—our best minds and our best work. As we get closer to control and elimination targets, it's helpful to consider the words of Dr. William H. Foege, who directed the US Centers for Disease Control, The Carter Center, and the Task Force for Global Health and helped lead the effort to eradicate smallpox:

> We don't do anything alone as individuals. Everything we do involves a coalition of some kind. . . . The difference is between coalitions that are just average and coalitions that are really great, and we have enough experience now to know what are some of the rules that make the good ones really great. And one of the rules is that you form your coalition around an objective, a last mile. . . . You don't form the coalition just because you have similar beliefs, or because you're a Republican or a Democrat or a Catholic or a Baptist. Because those kind of coalitions start out well, but then you get into arguments about where they should go.
>
> But if you can define the last mile, then anyone that signs onto the coalition knows where they're going. . . . With every program, there is a last mile, but then there are interim last miles. If you're going to drive from Washington, DC, to San Francisco at night, your last mile might be San Francisco, but you have a different goal for every state. And if you're doing this at night, you really can't see much, except what's in the headlights, and that's the way it is for many of our programs, that we can't actually see everything, but we have confidence, because of the last mile, that we know we're going in the right direction.

CHAPTER NINE

Strengthening Health Systems

The leaders of the Rockefeller Sanitary Commission had a fundamental disagreement. Some said the commission's purpose was solely the reduction of hookworm. Others saw hookworm eradication as a wedge for creating a local public health system. This debate echoes a century later, as the global health community decides how and where to allocate resources. Tackle specific diseases (known as "vertical programs")? Or strengthen health systems to support prevention and treatment for the entire range of primary and specialized health needs ("horizontal systems")?

"In 1986 or '87, I was giving a keynote for the American Public Health Association," said Dr. William Foege.

Just for fun, I went back a hundred years to see what they discussed at their annual meeting, and I was totally floored to see that the discussion was on vertical versus horizontal approaches to health. I thought that was a far more recent argument that revolved around global health, but then I got to thinking about, well, we have a hundred years of experience since they were arguing this. What actually happened? My conclusion was that every time we had a tool we used it, and every time we used it, the infrastructure became stronger for the next tool—and that the argument of vertical versus horizontal is a losing discussion, because it requires both. It requires strengthening the system to be able to use the next tool, and the next tool strengthens the system even more.

The NTD community struggles with how to effectively keep sight of its own goals while linking to broader agendas such as access to clean water and sanitation, maternal and child health, universal health coverage, and integration of education and economic development issues. Individual interventions, like mass drug administration, have focused efforts, created accountability, and driven results, but there is no escaping the other issues. Get specific or go broad? Disease or system? The answer is to do both, while constantly asking if the single piece complements the broader puzzle, and vice versa. In reality, vertical and horizontal approaches often happen concurrently, and progress is the line that zigzags between them.

■ ■ ■

I met Dr. Jacques Sebisaho in 2014 at Opportunity Collaboration, an annual conference that brings together people working on sustainable solutions to poverty. That year, the conference was held at a Club Med on the west coast of Mexico. A conference on poverty reduction held at a Club Med seemed strange, but the topic and the list of people gathering there were significant draws. Opportunity Collaboration doesn't allow PowerPoint presentations, panels, or business cards. Its stated objective is to create authentic connections in an "ego-free zone."

Sebisaho was born on Idjwi, an island in Lake Kivu, one of the African Great Lakes, between Rwanda and DRC. Technically, Idjwi is part of DRC, in the province of South Kivu, but its remoteness gives it a kind of autonomy. "This is the only place that, around the region—from Rwanda to Burundi, Uganda and South Sudan, Ethiopia, Somalia—has never experienced war," said Sebisaho. Idjwi is not only removed from conflict, but it is stunningly beautiful, with thick, lush, green grass and trees, set in one of the deepest volcanic lakes in the region. About forty-three miles long, it is home to almost 300,000 people.

Sebisaho shared some early memories of Idjwi. "Most people lived in huts, and we had a lot of food. We ate a lot of beans and green bananas mixed together, called *kifukama*." His father became mayor of Idjwi in 1960 when DRC became independent from Belgium. Having a small boat, he would ferry women in labor to the mainland. "I remember going to the shore and seeing women being loaded into the small boat and being taken to Bukavu [a city on the DRC mainland], where the hospital was located."

Sebisaho's family history in this clan-based, Havu-speaking Bantu region stretches back at least as far as the sixteenth century, when his ancestors arrived on Idjwi. One of them became Idjwi's king. "The king is the guardian of the traditions," Sebisaho explained, adding that when the crown passes to the next generation, the succession of power must be approved by the island's native Pygmies. "No matter how rich or important you become in the society, no one can be above the king. Any matter—like, if someone stole something from someone—the first person they go to is the king. Only when the king cannot solve a problem will he advise people to go to the court." An accession dispute in the early twentieth century was exploited by the Belgians, who colonized Congo in 1908. The result was two kingdoms in Idjwi, one brother ruling the north, the other brother ruling the south. Sebisaho's uncles, descendants of those kings, now rule the island, but the conflict was also passed down. "I would say for the last forty years, they haven't spoken," Sebisaho said. "The king in the north hasn't visited the south, [and] the one in the south hasn't visited the north."

In 1991, Jacques Sebisaho was attending a seminary school in Bukavu when a mandatory census was ordered to determine who was Congolese. Conflict between the Hutu and Tutsi peoples in Rwanda had begun in the 1950s, with Hutus killing hundreds of thousands of Tutsis in 1959 and 1963. Each massacre was followed by waves of refugees fleeing into neighboring Burundi, DRC, and Uganda, where groups organized and tried to negotiate their return. In 1990, one group—the Rwandan Patriotic Front—invaded Rwanda by force. The ensuing civil war lasted until a 1993 cease-fire, which was undermined by the assassination of President Juvénal Habyarimana a year later, sparking the genocide of Tutsis throughout Rwanda. Over the next few years, the violence spilled over Rwanda's borders into DRC.

"In 1991," Sebisaho recalled, "some Congolese believed that those Tutsi who came in 1959—whoever even had a drop of blood of Tutsi—should lose their citizenship." Based on appearance alone, people received a stamp on their identity card: Congolese or Rwandan (the latter, in this case, was shorthand for Tutsi). If you were identified as Tutsi, you were at risk for discrimination and could even be targeted to be killed. Looking at Sebisaho's mother and brother, the officer said, "You are obviously Congolese," and stamped their IDs accordingly. "You are Rwandan," he told Sebisaho. Despite their protests, the family could not reverse the decision. "This was the beginning of the discrimination," said Sebisaho.

Growing up, Sebisaho knew that he would either enter the priesthood or become a doctor. "I chose the easiest one," he said. "I went to seminary, but my lessons in seminary weren't easy for two reasons. One, it wasn't the holy place that I thought it was. We weren't supposed to give the leftover food to the poor community that was really destitute. And second, I was again considered as a Tutsi, and some people at the seminary were saying that they cannot be a friend to a Tutsi. I was really disappointed there, so I decided to enroll in medical school." Despite the political insecurity, Sebisaho managed to finish his bachelor's degree in biomedical sciences in 1995 and started medical school at the Catholic University of Bukavu. At one point, he was captured and tortured, and he nearly lost his life. He was forced to flee DRC in 1997 and finished medical school at the National University of Rwanda in 2002.

After graduation, Sebisaho and his wife, Mimy, relocated to New York City, where they raised their three sons. Mimy worked as a registered nurse at New York–Presbyterian Hospital / Columbia University Medical Center. But Manhattan was a world away from Idjwi, and Sebisaho felt pulled to return home.

He had an aversion to anything related to NGOs and the United Nations. From what he'd seen, NGOs didn't make a real impact on people's lives. He thought building a business would be a more sustainable solution. His dream was to build an eco-lodge, a resort that would attract people from throughout the region, and eventually throughout the world, to come to Idjwi to enjoy the peace and paradise he remembered from his childhood. An eco-lodge would also provide jobs for the villagers.

"I've gone through a lot psychologically," he said. "I was traumatized. I needed something to heal me. I needed to face some realities in my life. I thought maybe helping Idjwi could bring me that, give me that experience of facing the reality that I was trying to run away from."

During a 2005 visit he made to determine the eco-lodge's location, two Pygmy children died in a neighboring village. "That was hard. Very hard," Sebisaho said.

> I asked why they died. People said, "Because no one can touch us. Because no one can treat us." It came back to me that marginalization is a real thing. I look at myself, who has been marginalized because of who I look like. It didn't matter what we had, what my

father had accomplished, what school I'd done. But at least I had a chance. I could travel. I could have a different life. I looked at these people. They have nothing else. They don't even have an option. It was very, very difficult for me. . . . That same evening, we sat together and I asked them what they thought would be a great thing to happen. They said they needed an infirmary where they can be treated, like anyone else.

The Pygmy populations across Congo have faced systematic discrimination and marginalization for centuries by both local Bantu tribes and European colonizers. Their history includes various times of being enslaved, massacred, and, horrifically, even hunted down and eaten. Colonizers brought Pygmies to be displayed at the 1904 St. Louis World's Fair and at zoos. Today, these groups of African rainforest hunter-gatherers often continue to be denied schooling, health care, identity cards, and land ownership. The word "Pygmy" itself is controversial and considered pejorative by some, but at the same time it is used by some of the native groups as a convenient and accepted way to describe themselves. Sebisaho explained that "Pygmy" is the term used in French, but the people are called "Mbuti" or "Bambuti" in Swahili, and "Twa," "Batwa," or "Abatwa" in Kihavu (a language spoken in Idjwi and parts of the DRC mainland) and in Kinyarwanda (the official language of Rwanda).

Sebisaho encouraged the villagers to build an infirmary and said he would help them if all locals could be treated there, including the Pygmy community. Despite some initial protests, enough of the villagers realized that access to better health care would improve all of their lives. But, they said, they had no money. Sebisaho told them, "You have sticks. You have mud. We have a forest here, because my family owns this forest. You can come and cut sticks and you have the mud. Let's build it." The next morning, they built a basic shelter. "The following morning, I was seeing children. It wasn't really set up. It was not really organized. There were so many people showing up. But I had to leave the third day. I promised that I would come back. I spoke to my wife and I told her, 'I have a feeling that we need to postpone the eco-lodge and attend to people first.'"

With this rudimentary setup, Sebisaho began going to Idjwi twice a year. Mimy and their children sometimes joined him. One patient made a deep impression:

> I don't remember her name, but I still have her picture. I saw the mother coming with two children. All were severely malnourished. She said that she had lost children with big bellies. They had edemas everywhere on the legs. Big bellies, small thighs, big feet. And the mother was saying, "Can you please save my baby? Can you please save my baby?" The baby died. I think she had intestinal worms. She was severely malnourished, that's certain. We didn't have a microscope then, so that was just intuition. Malnutrition and intestinal worms, they go hand in hand. We gave them some anti-worm medicine, but that was not enough. With that cry from that mother and those eyes from that girl, and when I look at her picture, I feel so much strength. I feel, "Oh, we should keep doing this."

The Sebisahos kept returning to Idjwi. "Every time we left, there was nothing [there to help the people]," Sebisaho said. "So we hired two nurses, and they started seeing the patients." In 2008, they were able to build a more permanent hospital structure, full of light and set against rolling green hills; there are enough rooms for patients to wait to be seen comfortably, doctors' offices, inpatient rooms, and a maternity ward. They started a nutrition program, giving out fortified porridge twice daily to malnourished children.

Money remained scarce, however. From the United States,

Sebisaho was bringing large duffel bags stuffed with medicine and supplies—donated or collected from facilities where they had been discarded. But, Sebisaho explained, the green duffel bags looked military issued, and he was arrested at the border by guards mistaking him for a rebel. They took $400 from his pocket and beat him. When the Idjwi community heard what had happened, "they wanted to take revenge. I said, 'We don't need to take revenge.' " From now on, the villagers said, "every time you want to come here, please warn us. We'll wait for you on the shore so that we can carry things." After relating this, Sebisaho added: "The reason I'm giving this story, it's not to complain. It's to show how even terrible things have helped galvanize the community around the work and the importance of what we're doing together." He registered his organization as an NGO, taking for its name the Swahili word for peace: Amani Global Works.

But by the end of 2011, he was burned out. A cholera outbreak had killed numerous people on Idjwi. "It's too heavy on me now. I can't do this anymore," he said. "I needed to tell the community. They needed to continue on their own. We'll support them from afar. When I called them, they said, 'You can't do that.' They sold chickens and goats. The next week, they said, 'We got some money to continue.' It was $1,500. This was great, but for $1,500 you couldn't continue. In the meantime, my wife was asking colleagues at work if they knew any foundation that can support Amani Global Works." One colleague said, "You can't give up on this," and introduced them to the Segal Family Foundation, which agreed to provide the financial and strategic support that Sebisaho needed.

■   ■   ■

When Jacques Sebisaho and I met three years later in Mexico, the END Fund had already supported national NTD mapping in

DRC. I wondered if Idjwi had been included. From Sebisaho's description, it could have been overlooked. Back home, I checked mapping data, and Sebisaho asked his team to look at how many patients were coming to the hospital to be seen for NTDs. According to the DRC Ministry of Health's NTD mapping survey, groups of people from five representative sites in Idjwi had been tested for intestinal worms, schistosomiasis, and lymphatic filariasis. More than 84 percent of the people tested were positive for at least one of these NTDs.

"I was shocked to see that we had so many patients coming for intestinal worms and elephantiasis," Sebisaho said. "When I look back now, when I look at that girl who died, I realize she was severely malnourished. I suspect those worms were just eating everything she was eating."

"One cannot have experienced the war without having been impressed anew, and depressed, by the amount of parasitism in the world" began Norman Stoll's "This Wormy World" lecture. "Just how much human helminthiasis is there in the world?" Stoll asked, acknowledging that many in the audience might "warily scratch a mental ear and mull over a remark that ends 'where angels fear to tread.'" Stoll answered his own question with a global survey of known helminthic infections and more questions. Where were they? Approximately how many cases were there? Some of his examples are stunning: a 1924 study in Guam showed that "less than one per cent of the natives were *un*infected with hookworm, whipworm, or roundworm." More than twenty years later, Guam's situation had not improved, Stoll said, because "enough was not done, and what was done was not done well enough."

Idjwi in 2014 was not so different from Guam in 1924.

"There are, fortunately, signs that postwar this gloomy picture will be brightened," Stoll said.

I am also hopeful, but the picture is too often gloomy. On my first trip to Idjwi, in April 2015, during one of the morning feeding programs, I noticed small scars on some of the children's bellies. Through a translator, I asked if the kids could lift their shirts. Smiling, they obliged. Every single one had scars, between a half inch and two inches long. Some had dozens. Some had many, many more. "Is this a common practice?" I asked. Sebisaho translated my question to the mothers and village leaders standing nearby, who all lifted their shirts to show where, as children, they too had been cut.

Traditional healers often cut children's stomachs with razor blades, Sebisaho explained, to release the negative effects of the worms or anything else that is bad inside. Because the razors often aren't disinfected, children occasionally die from infection after this treatment. Sebisaho had been considering opening a room in the hospital for traditional healers, so at least they could learn sterile practices to apply to their long-held traditions. It was an ongoing debate within the hospital team whether this was a good idea.

In a meeting with the village elders, some people confided that they were trying to change this practice. It would not come easily. But perhaps holdouts would change their minds if the distended bellies of the kids went down, as the hospital team said they would, with deworming and more nutritious food.

"I worked in a remote area of DRC for seventeen years, followed by another eight in Kinshasa," said Dr. Adrian Hopkins, former director of the Mectizan Donation Program. "When I left, people said, 'You've made our children much more mischievous, much more naughty.' What they meant was: our children are much more *active*. When I'd arrived, the children just sat on the ground. A healthy 3-year-old doesn't just sit on the ground and do nothing, but that's what was happening because the children were malnourished. They were full of worms. The way they measured success was the fact that we made all the children naughty. So, I actually took that as a compliment."

■ ■ ■

With the END Fund's budget already stretched thin, I wasn't sure how we would take on Idjwi as a new program. Given its remote location and lack of infrastructure, Idjwi would be more expensive than our other projects in terms of cost per treatment (a common metric in the NTD world). Fortunately, I had met another person at Opportunity Collaboration. Jeff Walker is a philanthropist and author well known for his cross-sector approach to global health, finance, music, mindfulness, and education. When I shared my concerns with him, he offered not only to make a financial donation, but to reach out to his network and find others to join. He encouraged Sebisaho and me to think about how deworming could fit into a larger systems approach to tackling these diseases across the whole country. Could we create a model for others to replicate? The Walker Family Foundation, the Vitol Foundation, the Greenbaum Foundation, Alan McCormick of Legatum and his family, and (again) the Segal Family Foundation stepped in to support this initiative.

Our first move was to remap for intestinal worms and schistosomiasis. We wanted to get a more granular look at the distribution of disease prevalence and intensity, to test more sites, and to establish a more robust baseline.

Deworming programs and other MDAs frequently take place in schools because the location inherently provides a structure for drug distribution (record keeping, a captive audience, assistance from teachers) and because schistosomiasis and soil-transmitted helminths disproportionately affect children in the 5- to 15-year age range.

To remap in Idjwi, therefore, we had to determine where the schools were. We needed to know how many children were on the island and how many schools would be included in the MDA program. "When we went to the Department of Education," Sebisaho recalled, "they told us there were 186 schools on Idjwi island."

> [In July 2015] we mapped everywhere using GPS tagging, every single village from the north to the south. What we found out: that there were actually 242 primary schools. To find the schools, we had to go to each village and ask village chiefs and other people where they thought the schools were. We had four motorcycles, and we sent two people to the north and two people to the south. At the end of each day, we would convene and talk about the schools we had seen and especially the schools that weren't known by the government.

"The biggest challenge that we had were the roads," recalled Dr. Michel Mudekereza, medical director for Idjwi Hospital. "Most of the roads in Idjwi weren't that practical, and most schools were inaccessible. Sometimes we'd leave the motorcycles downhill and walk a few miles because even the motorcycle could not reach the places where the schools were."

The data on school numbers and locations were sent to Dr. Maria Rebollo, an NTD mapping expert who had assisted with mapping DRC during her time at the Centre for Neglected Tropical Diseases at the Liverpool School of Tropical Medicine and who now heads the WHO NTD initiative, ESPEN. She chose thirty schools for the volunteers to return to for stool samples. These samples would need to be processed at a lab within twenty-four hours to determine the diseases' prevalence (whether they were present at all) and intensity (to what degree and severity they were present). Warren Lancaster, senior vice president at the END Fund, encouraged Sebisaho to reach out to NTD leaders in Rwanda who had mapped their country a few years prior. Two people from the Rwandan Ministry of Health—Dr. Irenee Umulisa, then director of the Neglected Tropical Diseases and Other Parasitic Diseases Unit, and Eugene Ruberanziza, an NTD technical advisor—brought ten lab technicians to train their counterparts in Idjwi.

I asked Umulisa if there were any other examples of the Rwandan Ministry of Health collaborating with DRC on this kind of project. "Oh, no," she said. "This is unheard-of." Most of the Rwandan team had never been to DRC—let alone Idjwi—even though it was right across the border. "There's never been any partnerships like that," said Sebisaho. "That was the first time."

In December 2015 at each of the thirty schools, eight girls and eight boys were chosen and given a lesson on NTDs. Then, stool samples were collected. In a temporary lab at the Idjwi Hospital, a microgram of feces was spread on a slide and examined under a microscope. Each worm can lay thousands of eggs per day; lab techs are trained to recognize the various shapes as hookworm, roundworm, whipworm, or schistosomiasis. The techs have four handheld counters, one for each type of worm egg, to tally how many eggs are observed per microgram, a number that determines the intensity of infection. If they reach a thousand, they can stop counting. A symphony of ticking and clicking sounds filled the room. There was hardly a sample that wasn't teeming with eggs.

"It was a big surprise," said Mudekereza, "and there was also a sense of hope, knowing that we knew the intensity and the prevalence, and so we could easily treat them."

In Kenya, mapping had led to clear targets: not everyone needed to be treated. But on Idjwi, almost everyone was infected. Everyone needed treatment.

"Initially, we only had 200 community workers in the north," Sebisaho said. "They weren't doing much because we didn't have enough funds to support them or send them out. For the sake of NTDs, the distribution, in order for us to cover the whole island, to go beyond the northern part of the island, we had to select and hire 300 more for the south."

Three days before the first MDA, teachers and health workers were trained by representatives from DRC's Ministry of Health. Then they went to the schools serving as MDA sites, nine in the north and twelve in the south. Even with so many challenges—rough roads, more schools than expected, not enough lab techs, inaccurate population data—the teams mapped and provided treatment across the entire island.

A permanent solution to NTDs on Idjwi will be a complex matter of treatment, changing cultural norms, improving overall health, and supporting economic development. But more than 200,000 children and adults received medicines for intestinal worms and schistosomiasis that first year, with the support of hundreds of community health workers and teachers. A new generation of doctors and nurses was trained on how to detect and treat NTDs. Village chiefs and religious leaders now understand the long-term impact these diseases were having on their community.

The kings from the north and south—Sebisaho's uncles, who hadn't spoken in decades due to their old rivalry—came together for the MDA. The governor of the state of Kivu, who, according to Sebisaho, hadn't been to Idjwi before, also came. He wanted to see how the program could be expanded across all of South Kivu. "It was a huge, huge celebration," Sebisaho said. On the one hand, he remarked, this work is about delivering medicine. On the other hand, it is "bringing communities together and bridging worlds."

■　■　■

"The making of permanent gains against this infection has come up against the changing of deep-seated, long-established customs that are not to be easily disestablished, and against nutritional and economic problems not to be quickly resolved," said Stoll. He quoted Bailey K. Ashford, who launched the first successful hookworm campaign in Puerto Rico: "Parasites plus poorly balanced food bring fatalities and serious grades of anemia which would not occur from parasites alone. . . . Only when the fundamental thing is done will the disease as a disease disappear from Puerto Rico. And that fundamental thing is the provision of better food. . . . It is, therefore, no longer a medical problem, but a sociologic one of the very first water."

Deworming will not solve all of Idjwi's ills. Infant and maternal mortality rates there remain some of the highest in the world. Access to family planning services is practically nonexistent. But for Sebisaho, the NTD program has provided a model that can be repurposed. With additional training and funding, the community health workers could distribute other medicines and offer other public health services. They could be educators on hygiene and sanitation; they could watch for signs of serious illnesses and refer patients to more specialized care. Meanwhile, Amani Global Works is now connected to the DRC Ministry of Health's national NTD program. Sebisaho is working vertically *and* horizontally at the same time. He said that before embarking on the NTD program, he hadn't been to DRC's capital, Kinshasa, before; now he has gone several times and is in closer coordination with the federal Ministry of Health.

After the first deworming day in Idjwi, I went house to house in one of the villages to check on some of the kids who had received treatment. A group of them ran out to greet me. I asked, through a translator, "Did anyone poop out any worms yesterday?" After a fit of giggling, they nodded yes.

"How big were the worms?" I asked.

One boy raised his two pointer fingers, holding them about a foot apart. With a grin, a girl pointed to the ground where there was a roundworm souvenir that she had saved.

Sometimes progress is measured in the smallest of ways, worm by worm.

CHAPTER TEN

The Last Twenty Centimeters

"Just like baking cookies but a little bit more sterile and a little bit more technological" is how Ken Gustavsen, executive director of corporate responsibility at Merck Sharp & Dohme (MSD), described the process of manufacturing ivermectin. Powdered raw material is mixed and pressed into tablets, which go into bottles and then "down the belt and into a crate." From MSD's manufacturing facility in Haarlem, the Netherlands, the bottles are shipped to a distribution center in Mirabel, France, and from there flown to the countries that participate in the Mectizan Donation Program.

In 2017, MSD Haarlem produced 840 million tablets, which reached 300 million people. Still, the production process is constantly being fine-tuned. "Right now, the Mectizan tablet is a three-milligram tablet," Gustavsen said. "When the program started, it was a six-milligram tablet. But the feedback we got from the field was that a person might need three milligrams or six milligrams or nine milligrams or twelve milligrams. If somebody needs three or nine, they have to break this tablet in half. It makes the dosing hard. We said, 'Great. We will go back, reformulate, do the stability studies, redo the tableting line, and change it from a six-milligram to a three-milligram tablet.' That's what we did."

Feedback also led to improvements in the packaging. "Mectizan was initially packaged in a foil pack. But the feedback from the countries and the NGOs was: if we want to treat a thousand people in a community, we have to keep pushing these tablets out [to remove them from the foil pack]; it's not really practical. We determined that making a bottle of 500 tablets would be a much more useful way to get the product in the field. Coincidentally, it also cuts down on waste. It's much more efficient."

Newcomers to the world of neglected tropical diseases often think that if the right pills could get to everyone with an NTD, the suffering caused by these diseases would end. That idea is based on the kind of order and logic displayed in a facility like MSD Haarlem, where outcomes are predictable and resources are available to optimize efficiency. But the NTD solution depends on far more than medicine. And drug delivery is actually quite complicated.

■ ■ ■

In September 2016, I visited Zimbabwe's National Pharmacy (NatPharm), a generic white building in an industrial neighborhood in Harare, where pharmaceutical drugs under the purview of the Ministry of Health and Child Care (MoHCC) are held after they've cleared customs and before they are taken to provincial and district-level health centers. A series of meetings had brought me to Zimbabwe, and I was planning to visit two MDAs, one a school-based deworming program, the other a new program for LF, which, with trachoma, had been added to Zimbabwe's NTD program just that year.

Coincidentally, the day I visited NatPharm, representatives from the International Trachoma Initiative (ITI) were inspecting the facility, the final step before starting azithromycin donations. The country's inaugural trachoma treatment program was going to start in the heavily affected Binga District. ITI was planning to donate $4.7 million of azithromycin. The END Fund would underwrite the cost of distributing medicines; training nurses (in Zimbabwe, unlike most countries in Africa, only nurses can deliver NTD medicines) and those supervising, monitoring, and reporting on the MDA; creating promotional materials and printing treatment registers; transporting and paying everyone (including money for air time on their mobile phones); and, after the MDA, managing and processing the data.

ITI's supply chain manager, Carla Johnson, along with two co-workers and the NatPharm representatives, invited me to observe the inspection. Before a country is approved by ITI, it must demonstrate that its management system is professional enough to receive and not lose the drugs, that its supply chain can deliver the medicine, and that there is funding from or partnership with either the MoHCC or other organizations, in this case, UNICEF, World Vision, and the END Fund. ITI had sent a test shipment of three pallets of the pediatric oral suspension of azithromycin and now was checking to see if the drug had reached its destination (it had) and what bumps it had encountered along the way. How long had it taken the pallets to get from point A to point B? Who touched the drug along the way? How long did the shipment stay in customs? Was anyone asked to pay a tax? (Drug donations shouldn't be taxed.) ITI had been to warehouses at the provincial and district levels. NatPharm was the inspectors' last stop.

Zimbabwe's MoHCC had started the application for the donation two years prior. The first hurdle was mapping to determine where trachoma was and was not. Sixteen districts had been mapped in 2014. The Global Trachoma Mapping Project had decided not to map the remaining forty-seven districts based on its data, which predicted a low probability for endemic trachoma in those regions. The MoHCC preferred to map the entire country but at that moment didn't have the funds to do so.

With endemic regions identified, the MoHCC had then explained to ITI its downstream logistics, including how the medicine would move from NatPharm to regional warehouses to district health centers, what the in-country transportation budget was, how the reverse logistics (e.g., leftover medicine) were handled, how empty bottles were disposed of, and what happened to expired medicine. Other ITI concerns: Was the drug registered in Zimbabwe as azithromycin or Zithromax? Documents such as certificates of donation, pro forma invoices, packing lists, and bills of lading would be sent electronically; were original copies required? In short, before sending the test shipment, ITI had needed to know that Zimbabwe had the capacity to receive and distribute millions of pills.

In public health, "capacity" means having both qualified people and the ability to execute a plan. Countries can lack capacity because their infrastructure is weak (e.g., their roads are rough, dirt, marked with potholes), because of political strife or fuel or funding gaps, or because they don't have adequate health facilities with the supplies and equipment to make them functional. Countries may lack human capacity: there may be shortages of trained health workers, a lack of specialized knowledge, or government budget shortfalls leading to months going by without health-care workers getting paid, creating a dwindling incentive to show up for work. Many developing countries face the problem that once people receive the highest level of training in their fields, they tend to concentrate in the capital cities, leaving gaps in rural health care; sometimes, they leave their home countries for better opportunities elsewhere.

In 2016, Zimbabwe was still emerging from decades of political and economic upheaval. Once known as the "bread basket of Africa" for its abundant agricultural output, the country in recent years had seen tremendous turmoil, which had begun with excessive government payments to veterans of the Zimbabwean War of Liberation, the conflict that led to independence from Great

Britain. The massive payments had been followed by a disas-trous 1997 land redistribution program, which seized farms from white commercial farmers, and a 2008 indigenization law requir-ing that 51 percent of any business be held by indigenous (i.e., black) Zimbabweans. Foreigners divested, while displaced farmers were taken in by neighboring countries. Basic resources like fuel, food, medicine, and potable water became scarce. The treasury was drained. In 2008, the low point, the country's hyperinflation reached 79.6 billion percent, and there was an outbreak of cholera. Since then, Zimbabwe has been trying to rebuild, but progress has been slow and unsteady. It adopted the US dollar as its currency and began to reconstruct its collapsed health-care system. And in 2012, Zimbabwe took its first steps toward a nationwide NTD program by launching a plan to treat and prevent eight NTDs: intestinal worms, schistosomiasis (known there as bilharzia), LF, trachoma, leprosy, rabies, anthrax, and human African trypano-somiasis (sleeping sickness).

■ ■ ■

At NatPharm, the warehouse managers, clad in blue coveralls, gave us a tour. Not designed to be a warehouse, the building was too small for what it needed to hold. There were boxes upon boxes upon boxes, some stacked so high they were precarious towers and seemed about to fall over. In some places, the cartons were up against the wall or on the floor, not on the requisite pallets, which prevent moisture from seeping into the boxes. Paths between the stacks were narrow and winding. The managers apologized for the overflowing condition. They recognized the need to build another warehouse. "The plans are ready," they said. As of early 2018, progress had been made on preparations, including funding, but construction had not yet begun.

The managers were performing their duties without enough space or enough people. When large shipments of medicines arrived simultaneously, the managers struggled to log, sort, and distribute them in a timely way. When transportation funding fell short, one drug would hitch a ride with another—which seemed to be efficient, except when waiting for the drug with funding to arrive could jeopardize the unfunded drug's shelf life.

"How do you keep track of expiration dates?" an ITI rep asked.

"We track on this Excel database," a manager replied. "We look through, line by line, to make sure the medicines with closest expiration dates are used first." He showed us the program, admitted that this wasn't an ideal system, and said he hoped the new warehouse could implement automated tracking.

For a drug like praziquantel, which is used to treat schistosomiasis, the clock starts ticking the second it leaves the manufacturing line: two years until expiration. Made in Mexico, it is shipped on ocean-going vessels and takes up to six months to reach Zimbabwe. Given that MDAs happen only once or twice per year, praziquantel's remaining eighteen-month window is tight. A stark reminder of how easily drug donations can go wrong lay before us in a cordoned-off area where expired medicine waited to be destroyed.

The ITI reps said that occasionally countries don't pass the review, but mostly the inspection process helps countries identify areas for improvement. ITI is strict—at $33 per treatment, azithromycin is one of the more expensive donated NTD drugs, and unlike other donated drugs, it can be used widely as an effective antibiotic to treat more than just trachoma. Multiply that treatment cost by tens of millions of tablets a year, and it's reasonable that ITI wants to make sure its donation arrives in the hand of someone at risk for trachoma—and isn't lost or sold on the black market, or doesn't hit its expiration date while waiting to clear customs. These real possibilities thwart the seemingly straightforward connection between pills, people, and the end of NTDs.

■ ■ ■

Launching the NTD program "was really difficult at the start, because we were just coming out of the crisis, and none of the partners believed in us," said Dr. Portia Manangazira, director of epidemiology and disease control at Zimbabwe's MoHCC. "I'm happy that we have managed to convince the partnerships that are around us, and also ourselves, to continue doing this work."

Manangazira was one of several speakers at a breakfast event the day after the NatPharm visit. Some of Zimbabwe's NTD players (MoHCC, Higherlife Foundation, Econet Wireless, the END Fund) were meeting the Harare hub of Global Shapers, a worldwide network of millennials dedicated to economically and socially benefiting their countries and communities. I had first met a group of Global Shapers at the World Economic Forum a month prior, including a Mongolian woman who was reforming road safety laws in her country and a Colombian man who was finding ways for the newly signed peace deal to be implemented at a community level. Before my Zimbabwe trip, I had reached out to Andrew Makonese, a teacher and "curator" of the Harare Global Shapers hub, and told him about NTDs. "If it's a problem for Zimbabwe, it's a problem for me," he responded—and offered to gather the group.

For the Global Shapers at the breakfast, learning about NTDs was a revelation. They understood immediately the severity of the situation and their power and responsibility in ridding Zimbabwe of the diseases. As millennials, they were a large segment of the population—and therefore were likely to be affected by NTDs. Investing in NTDs was investing in their future. "Our parents put HIV and malaria on the map," Gerald Chirinda later said to me.

"We need to do the same for NTDs." He jumped into the cause, making television appearances, writing articles and blogs, and engaging with Global Shapers throughout Africa.

This breakfast meeting and these connections between groups, between generations, were quite appropriately taking place at one of Higherlife Foundation's offices, a suburban house that had been the home of Higherlife's founders, Strive and Tsitsi Masiyiwa. One of their companies, Econet Wireless, is Zimbabwe's largest mobile telecommunications company (in 2016, the company had 9.1 million subscribers out of a population of 14 million: 65 percent of the country). "It was on the living room couch over there that we sat down and said, 'We need to do something more for this country,'" Tsitsi's sister, Petronella Maramba, told me before the presentations began. In 1996, with thousands of people dying of HIV/AIDS, Higherlife was conceived in order to give orphaned and vulnerable children scholarships for primary, secondary, and university education. Over the years, Higherlife expanded to include technology in education and health, and it now operates in multiple countries across Africa and beyond.

Despite the country's difficulties, the Zimbabweans I know are proactive optimists with the highest regard for education. Many of them hold multiple advanced degrees, all express a deep personal responsibility for moving the country forward—and there is hardly a better example than the Masiyiwas. A few days after I was introduced to Strive at the 2012 Conrad N. Hilton Humanitarian Prize dinner, he emailed to say he wanted to help the END Fund. He started with a $100,000 donation to support our work in Zimbabwe.

Later I got to know—and came to deeply admire—Tsitsi (who now sits on the END Fund's board) and learned about Higherlife's scholarship program. At first I thought it benefited hundreds, perhaps a thousand, students. Actually, the scholarship program directly supports tens of thousands of students, and Higherlife's online education platform is used by more than half a million students. The Masiyiwas think big for Africa's future. Tsitsi once mentioned that she and Strive support the US Holocaust Memorial Museum and had been on the museum's learning trips to genocide sites around the world. I was curious how they came to choose this cause out of the many possible focus areas for their philanthropy and activism. She said, "If genocide ever arises again in Africa, we want to be trained to detect the early signs and hopefully help prevent it. We feel it is our responsibility."

Econet Wireless partners with the MoHCC to send messages with MDA dates and disease information to cell phone users in areas that are to receive NTD medicines. When cholera broke out, Econet successfully sent health messages. Now it could overlap cell phone tower locations with disease prevalence and treatment maps. At the time of my visit, dates and information about the upcoming MDA had been sent to more than 4 million people. A typical message read: "Has your child been protected against bilharzia and intestinal worms? Schools and clinics will give free treatment and information from 26 September–1 October."

"For some reason," Manangazira said, "people believe that if something is put on SMS, it's authentic. They will drop everything and go to the clinic if the message says so."

■ ■ ■

After I returned to the United States, Carla Johnson wrote to say that ITI had approved Zimbabwe's application. As promised, she sent me sample ITI inspection forms: Azithromycin Test Shipment Assessment Protocol, Customs Clearance Guide, Storage Facility Inspection Guide, and New Country Discussion Guide (Supply Chain).

"We are not here to conduct a supervisory visit and we are

not evaluating your personal performance on the job," reads part of a sample introductory script. "Please feel free to speak frankly with us."

What does it mean to "speak frankly" about NTDs?

"You cannot talk about the disease without understanding that these are people who sometimes have to go ten kilometers for water," said Mwele Malecela. To speak frankly about NTDs is to put them in context. Dr. Adrian Hopkins, who treated neglected tropical diseases in Africa starting in the 1970s, described his first Mectizan MDA in the Central African Republic. Wanting to gauge the local population's knowledge of river blindness, he asked if they knew anyone who was blind. "That was my first big cultural mistake," he said. "You are not supposed to talk about blindness. Even someone who was sitting next to someone who was blind would say they have never seen someone who is blind."

To speak frankly about NTDs is to speak about poverty. "You would want the person to swallow the drug after a meal," Manangazira said, "but some households don't have a meal for days." Zimbabwe's school-based feeding program is intended to bring children in, with the hope they will stay—for both classes and the deworming program.

To speak frankly of NTDs is to see the effort to end them as a long-term investment, not a quick fix. The first three years Hopkins worked in Congo, no one listened to him. They saw him as a tourist doctor. But he stayed and earned their respect. "When you come back, and they see that you're genuinely concerned about their health, that's when you can begin to make an impact," Hopkins said. "You have got to be with the communities. You have got to understand the communities. You have got to learn how things go."

To speak frankly of NTDs is to understand that the diseases have been around for thousands of years, but not necessarily where they are now or where they will be. In Zimbabwe, Manan-gazira said, "way back, we never used to see trachoma cases, because at every household the safe water coverage and sanitation in urban areas was way above 90 percent." In 2014, an outbreak of schistosomiasis was reported in Corsica and mainland France, decades after the disease had been eliminated in Europe.

Sometimes to speak frankly of NTDs is to use not words but a picture. Zimbabwe's public awareness campaign for the LF program included widely distributed posters with an explicit picture of a very enlarged scrotum as an example of elephantiasis. I questioned the choice to use this picture but had to acknowledge its effectiveness. At the MDA, several men said, "We saw the picture, so we decided to take the medicine."

■ ■ ■

The LF MDA took place beneath a tree at the Doonside Farm in the Zvimba District in Mashonaland West, a few hours outside Harare. Many of the men, women, and children came on a big trailer pulled by a tractor. Others walked or rode motorbikes. Plowed fields stretched out around us, punctuated with trees. In the distance rose low hills. Several women had babies strapped onto their backs. Their clothes were a mix: some bright, boldly patterned wraps, some jeans, some shirts with logos like Aéropostale.

Treating LF means treating the entire community—adults and children. They arrived, gave their names and ages to the two nurses filling out intake forms, and then gathered to listen to a public health official explain (in Shona, translated for me by one of the nurses) that they were going to be treated for LF. The drugs they would take were DEC and albendazole.

The crowd lined up and swallowed their pills with sips of water from a tin cup. The nurses recorded who took how many pills. The first batch of recipients left and were replaced with another trailer's worth of people. For hours, as word spread throughout the area, people arrived at the tree, listened to the public health official, recorded their names, took pills, and went back to work in the fields.

Later we drove to the Wilderness Farm, whose workers were unable to leave the fields. We parked by the side of the road. The farmworkers walked over, gathered around the back of the truck, listened to the public health official, gave their names to the nurses, took the pills, and returned to their work.

. . .

The Madamombé School in the Seke District, an hour east of Harare, had concrete floors, a block of latrines marked for girls and boys, and a hand-washing station with soap. School-based deworming programs usually treat both schistosomiasis and intestinal worms, but the school had recently held an LF MDA, which had included albendazole. Since that drug also treats intestinal worms, on the day we visited students received only praziquantel for schistosomiasis.

A ceremony in the headmaster's office welcomed our entourage, which included representatives from the MoHCC, Higherlife Foundation, the END Fund, and Global Shapers. Village elders, some of whom had helped build the school, offered testimonies on deworming's positive impact. The schoolchildren wore smart uniforms with blazers and hats; the boys were in button-down shirts and ties, the girls in green and white gingham dresses. A few of the students addressed the crowd. "Most of us lacked focus in class," one boy said, "but now that the MDA program has come to our school, we are happy. A good body is a good mind." When a girl in her short speech said, "We thank you," she and her schoolmates bowed and curtsied on cue. Behind them, amid charts and notices that could be found at almost any school—assembly duties, school prefects—was the ubiquitous LF poster with the giant scrotum. A poster titled "Prevent Bilharzia and Worm Diseases" included a picture of a boy with roundworms coming out of his nose. It's true that during a fever, worms exit the body however they can, but this struck me as perhaps another unnecessarily graphic photo of a very severe case.

The walls of the classroom in which the MDA took place were crowded with bright, colorful posters: the numbers and months in Shona and English; local fruit, including mangosteens, jackfruits, rambutans, limes, persimmons, and pomegranates; parts of the body; parts of a tree; uses for water; types of sports and games; and the English alphabet, with upper- and lowercase letters: "aA, bB, cC . . ." Big yellow paper signs hanging from the rafters showed phonetic options: *sm* -ell, -all, -art, -ooth; *sp* -oon, -ort, -ell, -ade, -ear, -ider, -inach.

Two nurses ran the MDA. Throughout this week, seven teams of nurses conducted MDAs at two to three schools per day. The nurses went from classroom to classroom. One measured each child against a paper dose pole taped to the wall, then wrote the child's height and age on the child's arm. Based on that information, an assistant doled out medicine. The second nurse recorded names and dosages. In Zimbabwe, early childhood education is free, so children as young as 3 years old are in school and can partake in the school-based deworming programs.

■   ■   ■

In public health, the "last mile" refers to the last hurdle that has to be crossed before delivering medicines or goods to the most inaccessible areas. The "last mile" can also mean the final stage of bringing a disease to the point of control, elimination, or eradication. After the MDA, Chirinda and Higherlife's Kennedy Mubaiwa pointed out that there is the last mile, and there is the last twenty centimeters, the distance that a person's hand travels from receiving a pill to putting it in his or her mouth.

The pill starts in a manufacturing plant, travels across the world, checks in at NatPharm, and comes to a school, where it is handed to a student, who swallows it, soon excretes the worms, and returns to class. Many factors have the potential to wreck the effort—but they are outnumbered by the people around the world who are committed to winning the NTD fight: teachers, program managers, village elders, philanthropists, heads of state, parents, and health extension workers like Dasash Gebere in Ethiopia, who said it best:

> I have ambition to create a bright future for generations. I want to give kids and mothers healthy lives. I teach them how to prevent diseases caused by contaminated water and soil. Students approach me to solve their stomach issues, and I help them by providing medicine so that they don't miss school. It also makes them happy and lets them focus on their education. If the kid gets sick, he can't properly go to school. If the kid feels well, he'll get his full education. We need to follow up on this kind of change. It brings opportunity for students to attend school happily. I'm focused on the students' health system, and I want to give them a better future. I just consider them like my own kids or my sisters and brothers.
>
> I take care of them like that.

CHAPTER ELEVEN

Homegrown Philanthropy

Her Royal Highness, Queen Sylvia of the Buganda Kingdom in Uganda, delivered the keynote address at the 2017 African Philanthropy Forum (APF) in Lagos, Nigeria. "The development context is changing fast, as old relationships between the developed world and the developing nations are evolving into partnerships built around trade and business interests," said Queen Sylvia.

> In 1624, a well-known English poet by the name of John Donne gave us a phrase. He said, "No man is an island." And he went further to say that "I am involved in mankind." . . . Now, similar to the idea in John Donne's poem, and much closer to home, is the Pan-African concept of interconnectedness between all people. The Nguni language in South Africa calls it "ubuntu." . . . Ubuntu speaks to a unity that ties us to one another as members of the human race. Yes, it is a Pan-African concept, but it goes much further than that. It is a value that is found in just about every civilization on Earth, present and past. . . .
>
> The Archbishop Desmond Tutu in his memoir, *No Future without Forgiveness* (1999), describes ubuntu as a philosophy that says "my humanity is inextricably bound up in yours," that a person is a person through other persons. When we look at philanthropy, we are told the origins of the word lie in the Greek language, and that it means "love of man." Philanthropy is said to encompass a love of humanity in addition to harboring a sense of caring and

a deep desire to enhance or improve the human condition. It sounds very similar to ubuntu, doesn't it? It emphasizes community, connection, and caring.

Queen Sylvia is a twenty-first-century African monarch, a ruler of the largest ancient traditional kingdom in Uganda, and a global activist with degrees in economics and communications, who has worked for the United Nations. Her conviction that traditional leaders can improve lives across Africa led her to cofound the African Queens and Women Cultural Leaders Network, which launched in 2013 as a coalition of more than forty traditional leaders from sixteen countries. Queen Sylvia's emphasis on partnership was also heard in the words of Tsitsi Masiyiwa, who, in her role as the chair of APF's board, had opened the conference:

> Partnership collaboration is key in driving changes. . . . Governments can never solve all our problems. They were never meant to solve all our problems, and they never will have the capacity to do that. They have an important role to play, but they are not our saviors. The private sector is an essential driver of the economic engine of any nation and therefore has to play the relevant and strategic role that takes into account the local environment from which it operates. The challenges the African continent faces are too hard and too complex to be left to one player, so the private sector has to step in in a strong and very meaningful way. We need to get social issues discussed in board meetings as opposed to only making it an agenda for those who are involved in development.

Queen Sylvia noted that there are more than 165,000 high-net-worth individuals (those with personal fortunes over US$1 million) living in Africa, with combined wealth holdings of US$860 billion—"a proverbial gold mine," she said, while stressing the importance of consistent, organized giving rather than "quick-fix scenarios." Masiyiwa applauded the growing economies of Botswana, Côte d'Ivoire, Ethiopia, Ghana, Mozambique, and Rwanda, while urging the audience to "face the brutal facts about what . . . type of leader . . . we are now. . . . Let this be the start of a journey which will lead us, as philanthropists, to become more humble as leaders and more committed, especially in a financial sense, to bringing real change to our continent."

The African Philanthropy Forum—especially that year—was, as Queen Sylvia put it, "homegrown philanthropy." In 2017, after several years being incubated by the San Francisco–based Global Philanthropy Forum, the APF was for the first time operating as an independent entity with an all-African board and staff. The energy and ideas in the room made clear that Africans are at the forefront of shaping their own narrative and solving the toughest problems that face their continent.

The day after APF, the END Fund organized a program site visit for a group of board members and supporters, including Tsitsi Masiyiwa, William I. Campbell, Tope Lawani, and English Sall, a millennial American philanthropist. MITOSATH was created in 1996 after Dr. Francisca "Franca" Olamiju, during her youth service for the American NGO Africare, saw people immobile on a highway. "Why are they not leaving the road?" she asked her boss, who explained that they had lost their sight due to river blindness. Olamiju was unable to accept that so many people were blind simply because they lacked access to ivermectin. She became determined to fill that gap. MITOSATH now organizes mass drug administrations for river blindness, LF, intestinal worms, and schistosomiasis and also offers vitamin A and iron-folate supplement distributions. "The mission of MITOSATH is to support governments and to uplift the dignity of human life," Olamiju said. "Being healthy raises your dignity." An NTD, Olamiju explained, "is a silent killer. It won't kill the person immediately, but over the years, silently, it will."

The MDA we visited that day was not under a tree in a field, but in the urban slum Makoko. Years ago, the Nigerian government created this community with the idea of relocating and housing people with disabilities from throughout Nigeria who had been shunned by their local neighborhoods and migrated to Lagos. It had essentially become a neighborhood for the disabled. One Nigerian told me that all the disabled people living together like this made it easier for NGOs and volunteers to come by and help them by giving food or medical support. But to me, Makoko seemed like marginalization on top of marginalization. "The Destitutes Home" read a fading sign at the entrance. "Come, Donate and Give . . . God Will Help You."

In Makoko, thousands of people are packed together, living with open sewage and with garbage piled high and uncollected. Just walking around was difficult; the foul smell was overwhelming. A sign above a wooden shelter announced the "Chairman of the Lepers." The leader walked toward us enthusiastically to greet our group, shake hands, and introduce us to other members of his community whose lives and limbs have been impacted by leprosy. (Many people think of leprosy as a disease of ancient history, but still today there are about 200,000 new cases of leprosy every year.) The chairman's handshake was enthusiastic, but the feeling of his gnarled and missing fingers in my hand made a deep impression, like no handshake I had experienced before. We also met the leaders of the self-organized communities of the blind and the community of the maimed, and we were introduced to a group of people living with such advanced elephantiasis that their legs were swollen to at least five times their normal size. It felt surreal, unfair, overwhelming. But in the middle of it all, a mass drug administration was happening for deworming and treatment with ivermectin to ensure that no one else would suffer the effects of river blindness, elephantiasis, or heavy worm infections.

Rita Aizehi Aimiuwu, a Nigerian who founded the Amen Health Care and Empowerment Foundation in 2004 after working for WHO for more than thirty years, also joined us that day. At first, Aimiuwu had set up the Amen Foundation to provide basic medical care. Then, Amen expanded to include eye care (performing cataract surgeries and distributing glasses) and screenings for prostate, breast, and cervical cancer. With support from the END Fund, Amen began integrated treatment of NTDs on a mass scale in the northern Gombe State. Before the conference, I had spent almost a week with Aimiuwu in Gombe and saw her in action, convincing the emirs and other religious leaders of the region to support the distribution of medicines, boldly asking the governor of the state for more local financing to be invested in NTD programs, and overseeing an energetic staff working alongside the Ministry of Health to distribute medicines to millions of people.

With about 190 million people, Nigeria has 20 percent of the continent's population. Of these, 75 percent need treatment for at least one NTD. When the END Fund was first asked if we could help in Nigeria, we noticed that there were a lot of large international partners working there, supported mostly by USAID and DFID. But some of the smaller, local organizations weren't able to access funding. Their infrastructure was less sophisticated. We thought that this was a unique niche where we could help the smaller groups increase their outreach and achieve a higher level of technical proficiency. We also sought to engage and support more Nigerian leaders and advocates like Olamiju and Aimiuwu in the local fight against NTDs.

"A Nigerian would understand the context much faster and easier than people who are not conversant with the culture," Aimiuwu said. "That's one of the reasons I've been able to relate well with the emirs. I know the culture. I know what to say. I know what to do when I go to them. It's easy for them to accept me. It's easy for them to accept the program."

"When you get to a community," Olamiju explained,

the first thing you do is you go and notify the traditional rulers that you have arrived, and explain your mission. Once they buy into that mission, they will even tell you, "Come, treat my family first." The community people will be there when you're treating the leaders' families, and if the drug is good enough for their family, you can be sure that everybody will want to take it. But before the intervention, they will ask you to come, they will invite all the other subclan leaders, they will tell you, "okay, explain to them." They will ask you a lot of questions like, Why are you giving us this drug? What is the way forward? What is the solution? Do we have to pay for this? Once the community is well sensitized, compliance is high.

Community health workers go door to door to give NTD treatment. Aimiuwu and Olamiju also go door to door—to the offices of governors, senators, and religious leaders—to get local support from the community, which is a most sustainable, powerful way to secure local engagement.

Olamiju said that her inside knowledge of the culture empowered her to help bring change:

We realized that for schisto, there is an information gap. Children that urinate blood feel that it's part of being a strong boy. Just like females go through their cycles, the guys feel that they are becoming strong by being burdened by schisto. . . . They used to feel it was part of being a man. So, the paradigm shift was something we needed to do. It didn't happen easily. We had to go there, help, educate, show films, show documentaries. We used the school structure, their health teachers. Some of them set up health clubs. It took a while for them to realize that this is really a disease and schistosomiasis causes that.

A variety of media is used to explain NTDs: comic books featuring the character Bambu, radio jingles, posters, and what Olamiju called the "moonlight story." She told me of bringing people together at night to watch films, with the ulterior motives of drawing blood to screen for LF and slipping in an educational film about NTDs. "It's part of our culture to educate people. Once you call a disease what it is in the local language, it rings a bell," she said.

> Nigerians, once they are convinced that this will improve their health, they go for it. They want to hear about the solution. Nigerians are resilient to some extent. It makes them stomach a lot of things, which in this instance is not very good. If you are used to suffering, you probably forget that there is a solution and there is a better life. And that's where we come in. We are Nigerian, so we use that language. And the language is simple. It's just the truth. Say the truth. Tell people that there is a way out.

The same kind of commitment and local leadership is evident among many community drug distributors I have met in Nigeria and elsewhere. Umar, a drug distributor from Gombe, shared through a translator, "It was an honor to be selected. I understand that I'm contributing my share for my community. You do a good turn for people. One day, when it's your turn, they'll reciprocate."

∎ ∎ ∎

The staging area in Makoko where people waited to receive medicine was cramped and crowded, with hundreds of colorfully dressed men, women, and children lined up and chatting to each other and the MDA organizers. Community health workers carried megaphones to make announcements to the crowd and wore white shirts that said, "Elephantiasis? Take Mectizan and Albendazole." At the front of the line, a health worker stood with a tall, narrow, wooden dose pole painted green and yellow. If a person's height reached four dots, they got four tablets of ivermectin. If they only reached the segment with three dots, they received three tablets. Everyone also got one albendazole tablet. They swallowed their pills with a cup of water, their name was tracked in the register, and then the next person was waved up to the dose pole. One by one, children and adults took the medicines. This service was being efficiently provided in a square right in the center of the main shelters for the leaders of the lepers and the blind and maimed communities, with a backdrop of a large pile of trash. It was a professional delivery of one public health program—in an environment glaringly in need of so many others.

"I grew up in Nigeria," Lawani later remarked to me. "I know the reality in the open centers fairly well. But I have never seen, anywhere in Africa, that concentration of people who have been outcast by society for the reasons that this community has been. I just never actually have seen anything quite like that. . . . It's very good, because you're forcing yourself to not look away, which is what we in large, developing countries do. You're constantly looking away."

Walking behind Lawani and Masiyiwa during the MDA, I saw her look at him and say with a chilling clarity, "This is our generation's problem to solve." He nodded his head. Overhearing these words, I felt the intense weight of their responsibility. These two dynamic, powerful, creative African leaders were not shying away from their role in addressing the daunting challenges facing their continent. I was reminded of the rabbinic maxim: If not us, who? If not now, when?

■ ■ ■

The task of ending NTDs is complicated. While there are medicines and they are being donated, they must reach people who live in some of the most remote places in the world. Although

MDAs have sparked enormous progress, there are still hundreds of millions of people who have not yet benefited from the drugs. Others may be receiving medicine for some, but not all, of the diseases they are at risk for, so massive work needs to be done to scale up these effective programs. Treatment coverage must be consistently above a certain percentage to be effective. Donors and countries need to stay committed not only to the treatment phase, but also to the multiyear surveillance phase after treatment has stopped so that disease elimination can be certified. In the future, some diseases may develop drug resistance. And without improving an endemic region's water and sanitation, reinfection is highly likely for some of these diseases. While scientists have found answers to many NTD questions, the pathology is not yet entirely understood. Although treating NTDs is less expensive than many other health programs, hundreds of millions of dollars per year are still needed globally to reach these disease end goals.

Ending NTDs is complex. The solution requires the work and perspectives of numerous stakeholders. Transmission cycles, for example, depend on far-reaching and intersecting factors, from local customs to vector ecology to political will to the limited economic opportunities that leave people vulnerable to parasites and bacteria. War and climate change influence NTDs. Treating these diseases requires coordination of local, national, and global health systems. There are many participants—donors, NGOs, governments, aid organizations, public-private partnerships—each with its individual mission and priorities. Some argue for a vertical approach, targeting a single disease; others lobby for the broad improvement of health systems, including the infrastructure treating NTDs. Even when these diseases reach the elimination targets, ongoing surveillance will be needed.

But, perhaps most important, the issue of ending NTDs is simple. No person should suffer from any of these diseases. Their treatment and prevention can be (and, in many places, has been) accomplished through medicine and access to clean water and adequate sanitation. Ending NTDs brings health and wealth. Children stay in school longer. Adults are able to work more. In today's turbulent world, the movement to end NTDs has the tools, the partnerships, and a roadmap to dramatically improve the lives of more than a billion people. It can be done. It must be done.

Wherever you are, whoever you are, you can help end NTDs. How? Here are a few ideas.

1. *Raise awareness.* Talk to people about the diseases. Read another book—about NTDs, or about poverty, water, and sanitation, or about the effective altruism movement. Almost all of the people interviewed in this book have an online presence; you can find their research papers, articles, poems, letters, and books. If you are a student, write a paper about NTDs. If you are an author, write an article or blog. Post a story or video on social media. If you have family or friends in endemic countries, ask them about the diseases. Don't look away.

2. *Build local political will for addressing NTDs.* If you are from a country that has one or more of these diseases, advocate for more private and public domestic resources and attention to go toward tackling NTDs. Support a local NGO working on NTDs. Meet with your congressional representative, mayor, or governor, and share information on how ending NTDs can improve the economic, education, and health status of your community.

3. *Join the NTD effort professionally or as a volunteer.* Many types of skills and people are needed to end NTDs. There is a place for advocates, anthropologists, artists, entomologists, policy makers, political scientists, social media influencers, supply chain experts, vector control specialists, and much more. How can your ideas, hard work, imagination, research, voice, and talents contribute to this global movement?

4. *Help ensure that current NTD resources are protected and increased.* The US and UK governments are currently the largest international donors to NTD implementation efforts, but aid priorities and budgets are subject to change. If you are from one of these countries, make it known to your congressional or parliamentary representatives that you support ending NTDs as a global good and an effective use of aid. Countries such as Belgium, Canada, Germany, and Japan (and others) have local NTD coalitions and would benefit from increased activism on NTDs. Regional and global banks dedicated to alleviating poverty and supporting development, such as the African Development Bank, Islamic Development Bank, and World Bank, have opportunities to do even more to end NTDs through grants and concessional financing.

5. *Donate to an NTD organization.* There is an entry point for every person, whether you are in elementary school, in the prime of your working years, or long retired. It costs about fifty cents per year to treat one person for all five of the diseases talked about in this book. If you donate one dollar, you have paid for two people to be treated. If you donate a thousand dollars, you have ensured that 2,000 people receive medicines. A million dollars improves the lives of 2 million people. TT surgeries, to ensure that someone with advanced trachoma doesn't go blind, cost about $70 each; hydrocele surgery costs about $100.

6. *Now that you've finished this book, give it to someone else or donate it to a school or your local library.*

ACKNOWLEDGMENTS

My gratitude for the creation and evolution of this book is deeply and inextricably entwined with my gratitude for everyone who has helped me enter into, learn about, and serve the global community working to end neglected tropical diseases. I continue to be astounded and inspired by all the people who have committed themselves so wholeheartedly to improving the lives of some of the most vulnerable and marginalized people in this world. With the brilliance, innovation, ingenuity, compassion, and drive of the thousands of people working to end these diseases—and their open arms and open minds to include others in these efforts—I have no doubt that getting to the end is truly possible.

I especially want to acknowledge the vision, commitment, leadership, and incredible support of Christopher Chandler, Alan McCormick, Mark Stoleson, and Philip Vassiliou of Legatum and Doug Balfour at Geneva Global, who founded the END Fund, gave me the honor of serving as its inaugural CEO, and have been pioneers in how the private sector and private philanthropy can be catalytic in ending NTDs. They have also been dear friends on this journey and a constant source of guidance and wisdom.

I am also profoundly grateful to William I. Campbell, who has chaired the END Fund since its founding. Bill has been unwavering in his dedication to NTDs and is an example of how to be an activist philanthropist; his heart seems to get bigger and more compassionate with every year I know him. Without Bill's mentoring, leadership, and networking and without the deep engagement of his entire family—Christine, Nora, Sarah, and Mia—the END Fund would never have been able to be of service across so many countries, in collaboration with so many partners, and to the hundreds of millions of people who have received treatment because of our work. I couldn't have taken and sustained this leadership journey without you, Bill.

The END Fund board has been the most committed, active, inspiring, and hard-working board I have so far had the privilege to work with. I have learned so much from each of them, and I am enormously grateful for their individual contributions to the END Fund and to the global NTD efforts: Nicolas Andine, Doug Balfour, Gib Bulloch, Robyn Calder, Bill Campbell, Michael P. Hoffman, Tope Lawani, Tsitsi Masiyiwa, Alan McCormick, Melissa Murdoch, Katey Owen, Scott Powell, English Sall, Rob Vickers, and Christine Wächter-Campbell. Huge thanks also to the committed, insightful, and ever-supportive END Fund Technical Advisory Council members: Alan Fenwick, Danny Haddad, Adrian Hopkins, Peter Hotez, Julie Jacobson, and Pat Lammie.

END Fund staff and fellows, past and present, have all labored with love, technical savvy, and a deep commitment to the vision of a healthier and more prosperous world and to the daily, complex, and often tiring work needed to make this vision a reality, one person and one partnership at a time: Molly Anderson, Elisa Baring, Diana Benton Schechter, Christopher Burrowes, Hannah Chang, Claire Chaumont, Jesse Coleman, Carlie Congdon, Cecilia Dougherty, Alessia Frisoli, Catherine Garces, Eve Gatawa, Jeff Glenn, Michael Greenberg, Mandy Groff, Tamera Gugelmeyer, Yayne Hailu, Heather Haines, Haydee Izaguirre, Kimberly Kamara, Kate Kelly, Warren Lancaster, Sara Laskowski, Sashi Leff, Frank Lei, Taylor Mann, Katie Douglas Martel, Sam Mayer, Courtney McKeon, Scott Morey, Sarah Marchal Murray, Fouad Onbargi,

Karen Palacio, Mercedes Pepper, Greg Porter, James Porter, Ana Gabriela Power, Mariah Ridge-O'Brien, Stephany Salazar, Ivy Sempele, Yael Silverstein, Alex Sveikauskas, Jamie Tallant, and Abbey Turtinen. In particular, Courtney, Diana, Elisa, Heather, James, Jamie, Kimberly, and Yayne contributed to making this a better book. Thank you to the entire END Fund team for making this journey together joyful, high impact, and transformational in so many ways.

And thank you to the Geneva Global team members who supported the END Fund from incubation to flying with our own wings, especially Doug Balfour, Louise Makau Barasa, Andy Bej, Collen Boselli, Lindsay Burns, Tom Ford, Caitlin Garlow, Lisa Grewe, Danielle Khordi, Ava Lala, Tina Maltas, Chris Miller, Alison Morse, Jenna Mulhall-Brereton, Alfred Mwenifumbo, Kasey Oliver, Mark Reiff, Karen Robinson, and Gene White. James Drinkwater, James Mattison, and Colin Webb from Legatum provided absolutely essential support in the early start-up days of the END Fund.

I am also deeply grateful to leaders of the extended Legatum family of organizations for their support, friendship, and invaluable advice on this journey: Nick Grono of the Freedom Fund, Caitlin Baron of Luminos Fund, Baroness Philippa Stroud of the Legatum Institute, and Georgina Campbell Flatter of the MIT Legatum Center for Development and Entrepreneurship.

Our partner organizations inspire, inform, and guide our work at the END Fund on a daily basis. Special thanks to the teams at Amani Global Works, Amen Health Care and Empowerment Foundation, Amref Health Africa, APOC, The Carter Center, CBM, the Centre for Neglected Tropical Diseases at the Liverpool School of Tropical Medicine, Children without Worms, ESPEN, Evidence Action, Global Alliance to Eliminate Lymphatic Filariasis, Global Schistosomiasis Alliance, Fred Hollows Foundation,

FHI360, Helen Keller International, International Coalition for Trachoma Control, International Trachoma Initiative, Kilimanjaro Centre for Community Ophthalmology, Last Mile Health, Light for the World, London Centre for NTD Research, London School of Hygiene & Tropical Medicine, Mectizan Donation Program, the MENTOR Initiative, MITOSATH, Neglected Tropical Diseases Support Center, Orbis, Organisation pour la prévention de la cécité, Partnership for Child Development, RTI International, Schistosomiasis Control Initiative, Sightsavers International, STH Coalition, Task Force for Global Health, UNICEF, United Front against Riverblindness, WaterAid, World Food Programme, and the World Health Organization. We are grateful for the many exceptionally committed government teams, at all levels and across many ministries, and the offices of presidents and first ladies who are leading the way in their countries to coordinate and deliver national NTD control and elimination programs.

I have been inspired and profoundly influenced by the growing coalition of donors and active partners who are committed to ensuring that neglected people and neglected diseases are neglected no more. Particular thanks go to Mona Hammami, Rabih Abouchakra, and Nassar Al Mubarak at the Abu Dhabi Crown Prince Court's Office of Strategic Affairs; Mohammad Al Ansari of the Al Ansari Exchange; Her Royal Highness Princess Lamia Bint Majid Al Saud of Alwaleed Philanthropies; John Damonti of Bristol-Myers Squibb; Sir Christopher Hohn and the team at the Children's Investment Fund Foundation; Strive and Tsitsi Masiyiwa of Delta Philanthropies; H. E. Tariq Al Gurg and the team at Dubai Cares; Robyn Calder, Tom McPartland, and the team at ELMA Philanthropies; Elie Hassenfeld and the team at GiveWell; Good Ventures; Melissa Murdoch and her family at Green Park Foundation; Tsitsi Masiyiwa, Bernard Chidzero, Kennedy Mubaiwa, and many others at Higherlife Foundation; Chuck

Slaughter at Horace W. Goldsmith Foundation; Walter Panzirer, Trista Kontz-Bartels, and the team at the Leona M. and Harry B. Helmsley Charitable Trust; Christine Morse, Paul Busch, Terrence Meersman, and the team at Margaret A. Cargill Philanthropies; Oxford University Press; Segal Family Foundation; Khaled and Olfat Juffali and all of the Shefa Fund investors;UBS Optimus Foundation; Vitol Foundation; Walker Family Foundation; Wallace Genetic Foundation; and hundreds of individual generous donors.

The support from leaders inside so many high-impact organizations that are committed to making the world a better place has also made this work possible: Africa Grantmakers' Affinity Group, African Philanthropy Forum, Bridgespan, Co-Impact, Global Citizen, Global Health Strategies, Global Philanthropy Forum, Legatum Institute, Opportunity Collaboration, Panorama Global, Sabin Vaccine Institute, Skoll Foundation, Speak Up Africa, Synergos, TED, Tri-State Area Africa Funders Group, UK Department for International Development, UK Natural History Museum, Uniting to Combat NTDs, US Agency for International Development, the World Bank, and the World Economic Forum.

None of the work described in this book would be possible without the generous drug donations from and phenomenally committed people working at Eisai, GlaxoSmithKline, Johnson & Johnson, Merck Serono, MSD, and Pfizer.

Exceptional gratitude goes to the many people I have had the privilege to work with at the Bill & Melinda Gates Foundation, without whom the END Fund and this book would not have been possible. I offer my particular thanks for invaluable support and guidance to Jennifer Alcorn, Hassan Al-Damluji, Simon Brooker, Don Bundy, Joe Cerrell, Bart Cornelissen, Meg DeRonghe, Sue Desmond-Hellmann, Alexandra Farnum, Max Gasteen, Catherine Goode, Kitty Harding, Erin Hulme, Julie Jacobson, Hannah Kettler, Nana Kwadwo-Biritwum, Edward Lloyd-Evans, Molly Mort,

Trevor Mundel, Katey Owen, Kendra Palmer, Rob Rosen, Mark Suzman, Jordan Tappero, Ann Varghese, and Rebecca Weber. The team at the foundation upholds its reputation: "impatient optimists" with a belief that "all life has equal value." Bill and Melinda Gates, thank you for showing us that the voices and resources of the most powerful can and should be used to stand up for and to improve the lives of the most vulnerable.

Enormous thanks also to the photographers, videographers, translators, and transcribers who have worked with the END Fund over the years to help us capture the stories of people on the front line of NTD work, many of which appear in this book: Funmilayo Adedotun, Jaad Asante, Menbi Awoke, Alexandria Bombach, Ora Dekornfeld, Jessica Dimmock, Sarah Ginsburg, Adey Hailu, Catherine Bell Johnson, Saskia Keeley, Meredith Lobsinger, Misgan "Mario" Assefa Lulie, Laura Martin, Rachael Missall, Jon Moe, Tinashe Njagu, Abbey Reznicek, Ryan Scafuro, and Mehari Worku. I'm especially grateful to the exceptionally talented Lindsay Branham and Jonathan Olinger, who joined and captured my first NTD field visit in Mali in 2012, and to Mo Scarpelli, who continues, with such insight and compassion, to ensure that the voices and views of those affected by NTDs are at the center of our stories. Thank you to Robin Coleman at Johns Hopkins University Press for believing that these stories need to be told and for supporting this book from idea through publication. My sincere gratitude to copyeditor Merryl A. Sloane for her impeccable work and gifted eye.

Heartfelt thanks to dear friends and advisors Jeff Walker and Sharon Salzberg, who provided so much personal support and wise counsel during the writing of this book—and indeed, through their example, helped me to see that it was possible.

Of course, this book could have never happened without the talent, creativity, drive, compassion, and insight of my coauthor,

Mojie Crigler. We truly have been preparing to write this book together for a lifetime, and one of the best gifts from this collaboration has been our deepened friendship. Finally, no thanks are enough for Jeff and Calissa; without your patience, flexibility, and support for my work and travel, none of this would be possible.

Much of the material in this book comes from interviews and conversations; the names of those individuals are listed under the relevant chapter headings below. Academic papers, newspaper articles, books, and online sources have provided further information. A central resource for understanding the diseases and the issues surrounding them is Peter J. Hotez's *Forgotten People, Forgotten Diseases*. Complete references are in the bibliography.

Chapter 1. Crisis and Collaboration

Most of this chapter is based on my own recollections of the 2012 regional consultative meeting for NTDs, the ensuing fundraising, and the October MDA. More details and information come from the END Fund's Warren Lancaster, Elisa Baring, and Heather Haines; Christopher Chandler; and Emily Wainwright of USAID. I reviewed transcripts of speeches given at a press event for the Mali mining companies, and HKI provided transcripts of the radio announcements. The Erasmus University study on financial gains from eliminating NTDs was reported in Redekop et al., "The Socioeconomic Benefit to Individuals of Achieving the 2020 Targets for Five Preventive Chemotherapy Neglected Tropical Diseases."

Chapter 2. Modern Approaches to Ancient Diseases

Anthony Solomon and Helen Bokea granted lengthy, enlightening interviews. Information on trachoma's transmission cycle, symptoms, old and new treatments, long-term complications, cultural history, and taboos is in Schlosser's "History of Trachoma" (prepared for the International Trachoma Initiative); WHO's September 26, 2014, "Weekly Epidemiological Report"; Sheila K. West's "Azithromycin for Control of Trachoma"; and Paul Courtright et al.'s "Women and Trachoma: Achieving Gender Equity in the Implementation of SAFE," a manual created by the Elfenworks Foundation, The Carter

Center, and the Kilimanjaro Centre for Community Ophthalmology. Additional information is on the websites of WHO, ITI, International Coalition for Trachoma Control, Sightsavers, Pfizer, The Carter Center, and the National Center for Biotechnology Information. Ji-Hye Shin's article "The 'Oriental' Problem: Trachoma and Asian Immigrants in the United States, 1897-1910" provides both data and insight. Dr. Youssef Chami Khazraji is quoted in Ruth Levine et al.'s *Millions Saved: Proven Successes in Global Health*, which offers a detailed account of Morocco's trachoma elimination campaign. The report of WHO's 1996 meeting, which set 2020 as the target year for the elimination of trachoma as a disease of public health importance, was published as World Health Organization, *Future Approaches to Trachoma Control: Report of a Global Scientific Meeting*. The interviews with Melese Kitu and Achenef Demilew were conducted by Mo Scarpelli and translated by Eskinder Temtme.

Chapter 3. Big Consequences from Small Things

Talking to William C. Campbell about ivermectin's origins was a highlight of writing this book. He also shared numerous documents that provided technical details, including a number he wrote: "The Genesis of the Antiparasitic Drug Ivermectin"; "Chemotherapy of Helminth Infections: A Centennial Reflection"; "Serendipity in Research Involving Laboratory Animals"; "In Memoriam: Ashton C. Cuckler"; "In Memoriam: James Desmond Smyth, Honorary Member, ASP"; and "History of Avermectin and Ivermectin, with Notes on the History of Other Macrocyclic Lactone Antiparasitic Agents." Additional information on ivermectin's early history can be gleaned from Austin, Barrett, and Weber, "Merck Global Health Initiatives (A)." Roy Vagelos generously explained the lead-up to Merck's decision to donate ivermectin. See also Dr. Vagelos's memoir, *Medicine, Science, and Merck* (with Louis Galambos); Michael Useem's "Roy Vagelos Attacks River Blindness"; and *New York Times* articles "Merck Offers Free Distribution of New River Blindness Drug" and "River Blindness: Conquering an Ancient Scourge" by Erik Eckholm. André C. Rougemont's letter was printed in the *Lancet* on November 20, 1982.

Daniel Boakye's memories of OCP and explanations of the complex black fly are invaluable. The World Bank's *The Onchocerciasis Control Program in West Africa* by Bernard H. Liese et al. provides essential data. Over two lengthy interviews, Uche Amazigo recounted the history of APOC and CDTI, and she made several excellent suggestions for further research. Her chapter, "The Development of Community Directed Treatment for Tackling River

Blindness," in Francis Omaswa and Nigel Crisp's *African Health Leaders: Making Change and Claiming the Future* is particularly helpful. Dr. Mona Hammami explained the history and strategy behind the Reaching the Last Mile Fund. Bahman M. Abdulredha offered reflections and information on Kuwait's long involvement in the fight against river blindness. John Coles's *Blindness and the Visionary*, F. C. Rodger's *Blindness in West Africa*, and Sir John Wilson's *Travelling Blind* illustrate Wilson's life and the early years of the organization that became Sightsavers. Lady Jean Wilson offered detailed recollections of her adventures and work with her late husband. During our interview, she recounted, "Helen Keller was a very good friend of ours. She'd come from Scotland and we'd meet her in Paddington. There was the lady, perfectly dressed, perfectly hatted, after sleeping on a train all night. She usually stayed at her daughter's home and people would send her flowers. She would go around and smell all the flowers, even the ones who had no perfume at all, recognizing the scent. Then she would come to one and say, 'This is the loveliest fragrance of all,' and that would be from me and John—pure Scotch."

Chapter 4. Empowerment and Humility

Mwele Malecela, David Addiss, Patrick Lammie, and Yao Sodahlon generously shared their experiences and expertise in addressing LF. More information is available in Malcolm Dean's *Lymphatic Filariasis: The Quest to Eliminate a 4,000-Year-Old Disease*; "Translating Research into Reality—Elimination of Lymphatic Filariasis from Haiti" by Patrick Lammie et al.; and David Addiss's "Global Elimination of Lymphatic Filariasis" and "Spiritual Themes and Challenges in Global Health." The interviews with Mitku Mengistu and Yealemwerk Emshaw were conducted by Mo Scarpelli with Misgan "Mario" Assefa Lulie interpreting. The transcript of Mengistu's interview was translated by Eskinder Temtme; Emshaw's was translated by Adey Hailu.

Chapter 5. Worms, Maps, and Money

The history of the RSC's hookworm campaign is drawn largely from *To Cast Out Disease* by John Farley; "Disease and Development: Evidence from Hookworm Eradication in the American South" by Hoyt Bleakley; and the trove of primary sources (including photographs amd silent films) in the Rockefeller Foundation's online archive (www.rockefeller100.org). *Parasites, Pathogens, and Progress* by Robert A. McGuire and Philip R. P. Coehlo provides information on hookworm's influence on slavery and the Civil War.

The literature on deworming's link to education is vast; I relied on "Worms: Identifying Impacts on Education and Health in the Presence of Treatment Externalities" by Edward Miguel and Michael Kremer; "Deworming" by Andrew Hall and Sue Horton; "The Challenge of Hunger and Malnutrition" by Sue Horton et al.; "Monitoring and Evaluating the Impact of National School-Based Deworming in Kenya" by Charles S. Mwandawiro et al.; *Exploiting Externalities to Estimate the Long-Term Effects of Early Childhood Deworming* by Owen Ozier; and Norris et al.'s *Social and Economic Impact Review on Neglected Tropical* Diseases, which was produced for the Hudson Institute in conjunction with Global Network for NTDs. Interviews with Simon Brooker, Don Bundy, Elie Hassenfeld, Michael Kremer, and Bjørn Lomborg greatly illuminated the many sides of the economic debate on NTDs. Don Bundy filled in the late twentieth-century history on school-based health and nutrition programs, and he suggested critical and fascinating literature, including chapters in the 1993 and 2006 editions of *Disease Control Priorities in Developing Countries*, and the article "Control of Geohelminths by Delivery of Targeted Chemotherapy through Schools" by Bundy, Wong, et al.

Chapter 6. A New Normal

Many people interviewed for this book discussed NTDs being unseen and regarded as a normal part of life. Chinyelu Ekwunife, Corine Karema, Dirk Engels, Matshidiso Moeti, and Uche Amazigo provided especially vivid, insightful descriptions of this mind-set and many other aspects of NTDs. Ekwunife, Okafor, and Mwaorgu, "Ultrasonic Screening of Urinary Schistosomiasis Infected Patients in Agulu Community, Anambra State, Southeast Nigeria," and Ekwunife, "Socio-Economic and Water Contact Studies in *Schistosomiasis* [sic] *haematobium* Infested Area of Anambra State, Nigeria," explain some of the challenges specific to this disease. Alan Fenwick was a tremendous resource on schistosomiasis's transmission cycle, mysteries, and vulnerability to praziquantel. Schistosomiasis's history in China is drawn from an insightful interview with Yaobi Zhang, as well as Frank A. Kierman Jr.'s *Harper's Magazine* article "The Blood Fluke That Saved Formosa" and Kawai Fan and Honkei Lai's "Mao Zedong's Fight against Schistosomiasis." The interviews with Simeon Ogola Aquiro and Boniface Opinya were conducted in English by Mo Scarpelli, who also interviewed Biruk Kebede Negash and Seifu Tirfie. Data on the necessary increased distribution of praziquantel come from World Health

Organization, *Report of the Tenth Meeting of the WHO Strategic and Technical Advisory Group for Neglected Tropical Diseases.*

Chapter 7. Stone Soup

Interviews with David Brandling-Bennett, Meg DeRonghe, Gabrielle Fitzgerald, Kitty Harding, Julie Jacobson, Katey Owen, and Regina Rabinovich painted the picture of the Bill & Melinda Gates Foundation's early years. W. Wayt Gibb's "Bill Gates Views Good Data as Key to Global Health" in *Scientific American* and Gates's own "Here's My Plan to Improve Our World—And How You Can Help" in *Wired* provide some of Gates's perspective. The 2012 London Declaration is available at https://www.youtube.com/watch?v=VQcXBrXPzjs. Data for the fifth anniversary are available at http://www.unitingtocombatntds.org/5th-anniversary.

Chapter 8. Unfrozen Moment

Interviews with Don Bundy, Alan Fenwick, William H. (Bill) Foege, Peter J. Hotez, David Molyneux, and Emily Wainwright greatly deepened my understanding of the NTD sector in the mid-2000s. Doug Balfour, William I. Campbell, Christopher Chandler, and Alan McCormick talked to me at length about Legatum's early NTD ventures and the creation of the END Fund. Further information comes from Institutional Investor's "Secrets of Sovereign" and Andrew Jack's *Financial Times* articles on NTDs. The Republic of Rwanda's "Mapping of Schistosomiasis and Soil-Transmitted Helminthiasis in Rwanda 2014"; CBM's "Proposal: Elimination of Blinding Trachoma in Burundi (2012-2013)"; Geneva Global's "Rwanda and Burundi Tropical Disease Control: 2007-2010 Report"; and Josh Ruxin and Joel Negin's "Removing the Neglect from Neglected Tropical Diseases: The Rwandan Experience, 2008-2010" provide data for Legatum's projects in Rwanda and Burundi. Additional data and details about the project in Rwanda came from interviews conducted by Mo Scarpelli with Jmu Mbonyiintwari and Irenee Umulisa. Tope Lawani described in detail his experience rediscovering NTDs and the myriad ways in which solving NTDs makes sense from a financier's point of view.

Chapter 9. Strengthening Health Systems

Conversations with Jacques Sebisaho, Warren Lancaster, Michel Mudekereza, and Irenee Umulisa augmented my recollections of Opportunity Collaboration and working with Amani Global Works in Idjwi. I draw on David S. Newbury's *Kings and Clans: Idjwi Island and the Lake Kivu Rift, 1780–1840* for information on Idjwi's societal structure. I have followed the suggestions at www.survivalinternational.org/info/terminology for the most respectful way to reference the Pygmies.

Chapter 10. The Last Twenty Centimeters

This chapter is based on my experience in Zimbabwe in 2016 and on conversations with Gerald Chirinda, Portia Manangazira, Petronella Maramba, Kennedy Mubaiwa, and Ken Gustavsen, who shared pictures and internal documents on the Mectizan Donation Program and MSD Haarlem. Carla Johnson was instrumental to my inside look at ITI's inspection process and provided me with forms, guides, and instructions. Information on NatPharm's new warehouse can be found at https://constructionreviewonline.com/2017/01/natpharm-constructs-regional-warehouse-in-zimbabwe. Chirinda's work is described in Beaven Tapureta's "Young Writers Show Africa the Way." Information on Zimbabwe's economic turmoil in recent decades is drawn from Steve H. Hanke and Alex K. F. Kwok's "On the Measurement of Zimbabwe's Hyperinflation." Information on Zimbabwe's NTD program comes from the Zimbabwe Ministry of Health and Child Welfare's "National Strategic Plan and Programme for the Control of Neglected Tropical Diseases, 2012–2016" and "Training Manual, 2012–2016: Mass Drug Administration (MDA) for Schistosomiasis (Bilharzia) and Soil Transmitted Helminths (Intestinal Worms)." Mapping data can be found at http://journals.plos.org/plosntds/article?id=10.1371/journal.pntd.0003014. Strive and Tsitsi Masiyiwa continue to give me an invaluable understanding of Zimbabwe and philanthropy. The interview with Dasash Gebere was conducted by Mo Scarpelli and translated by Eskinder Temtme.

Chapter 11. Homegrown Philanthropy

Her Royal Highness, Queen Sylvia of Buganda Kingdom in Uganda, and Tsitsi Masiyiwa spoke at the 2017 African Philanthropy Forum in Lagos, which I attended. Jeff Glenn provided vital insight into systems change and systems theory. Mo Scarpelli and I interviewed Rita Aizehi Aimiuwu, and Mo interviewed Dr. Francisca Olamiju and Umar. Funmilayo Adedotun translated Umar's words.

Addiss, David G. "Global Elimination of Lymphatic Filariasis: A 'Mass Uprising of Compassion.'" *PLOS Neglected Tropical Diseases* 7 (2013): e2264. https://doi.org/10.1371/journal.pntd.0002264.

———. "Spiritual Themes and Challenges in Global Health." *Journal of Medical Humanities* (2015): doi:10.1007/s10912-015-9378-9.

African Programme for Onchocerciasis Control and WHO. "Revitalising Health Care Delivery in Sub-Saharan Africa." 2007. In possession of author.

Amazigo, Uche. "The Development of Community Directed Treatment for Tackling River Blindness." In *African Health Leaders: Making Change and Claiming the Future,* edited by Francis Omaswa and Nigel Crisp, 125–43. Oxford: Oxford University Press, 2014.

Austin, James E., Diana Barrett, and James Weber. "Merck Global Health Initiatives (A)." Harvard Business School Case 9-301-088, January 2001. https://hbr.org/product/merck-global-health-initiatives-a/301088-PDF -ENG.

Balfour, Doug. *Doing Good Great: An Insider's Guide to Getting the Most Out of Your Philanthropic Journey.* Wayne, PA: Geneva Global, 2015.

Bleakley, Hoyt. "Disease and Development: Evidence from Hookworm Eradication in the American South." *Quarterly Journal of Economics* 122 (2007): 73–117. doi:10.1162/qjec.121.1.73.

Brooker, Simon, Peter J. Hotez, and Donald A. P. Bundy. "Hookworm-Related Anaemia among Pregnant Women: A Systematic Review." *PLOS Neglected Tropical Diseases* 2 (2008): e291. doi:10.1371/journal.pntd.0000291.

Bundy, D. A. P., C. Burbano, et al. *Rethinking School Feeding, Social Safety Nets, Child Development, and the Education Sector.* Washington, DC: World Bank Publications, 2009.

Bundy, D. A. P., S. Shaeffer, et al. "School Based Health and Nutrition Programs." In *Disease Priorities in Developing Countries*, 2nd ed., edited by
D. Jamison et al., 1091-1108. New York: World Bank and Oxford University Press, 2006.

Bundy, D. A. P., M. S. Wong, et al. "Control of Geohelminths by Delivery
of Targeted Chemotherapy through Schools." *Transactions of the Royal
Society of Tropical Medicine and Hygiene* 84(1) (1990): 115-20.

Campbell, William C. "Chemotherapy of Helminth Infections: A Centennial Reflection." In *A Century of Parasitology: Discoveries, Ideas and
Lessons Learned by Scientists Who Published in the "Journal of Parasitology,"
1914-2014*, edited by John Janovy Jr. and Gerald W. Esch, 202-14. West
Sussex, England: Wiley, 2016.

———. "The Genesis of the Antiparasitic Drug Ivermectin." In *Inventive
Minds: Creativity in Technology*, edited by Robert J. Weber and David N.
Perkins, 194-214. New York: Oxford University Press, 1992.

———. "History of Avermectin and Ivermectin, with Notes on the History of
Other Macrocyclic Lactone Antiparasitic Agents." *Current Pharmaceutical
Biotechnology* 13(6) (2012): 853-65. doi:10.2174/138920112800399095.

———. "In Memoriam: Ashton C. Cuckler." *Journal of Parasitology* 87(2) (2001):
466-67. doi:10.1645/0022-3395(2001)087[0466:IMACC]2.0.CO;2.

———. "In Memoriam: James Desmond Smyth, Honorary Member, ASP."
Journal of Parasitology 85(5) (1999): 992-93.

———. "Serendipity and New Drugs for Infectious Disease." *ILAR Journal* 46
(2005): 352-56.

———. "Serendipity in Research Involving Laboratory Animals." *ILAR Journal*
46 (2005): 329-31.

———. "Treatment under the Big Tree." MDP's *Mectizan Program Notes* 20
(1998).

CBM. "Proposal: Elimination of Blinding Trachoma in Burundi (2012-2013)."
October 16, 2011. In possession of author.

Cochi, Stephen L., and Walter R. Dowdle, eds. *Disease Eradication in the 21st
Century: Implications for Global Health*. Cambridge, MA: MIT Press, 2011.

Coles, John. *Blindness and the Visionary: The Life and Work of John Wilson*.
London: Giles de la Mare Publishers, 2006.

Courtright, Paul, Elizabeth Cromwell, and Paul Emerson. "Women and
Trachoma: Achieving Gender Equity in the Implementation of SAFE."

2009. https://www.cartercenter.org/resources/pdfs/health/trachoma
/women_trachoma.pdf.

Crisp, Geoffrey. *Simulium and Onchocerciasis in the Northern Territories of the Gold Coast.* London: H. K. Lewis for the British Empire Society for the Blind, 1956.

Dean, Malcolm. *Lymphatic Filariasis: The Quest to Eliminate a 4000-Year-Old Disease.* Hollis, NH: Hollis Publishing, 2001.

Despommier, Dickson D. *People, Parasites, and Plowshares: Learning from Our Body's Most Terrifying Invaders.* New York: Columbia University Press, 2013.

de Vlas, Sake J., et al. "Concerted Efforts to Control or Eliminate Neglected Tropical Diseases: How Much Health Will Be Gained?" *PLOS Neglected Tropical Diseases* 10(2) (2016): e0004386. https://doi.org/10.1371/journal
.pntd.0004386.

Drisdelle, Rosemary. *Parasites: Tales of Humanity's Most Unwelcome Guests.* Berkeley: University of California Press, 2010.

Eckholm, Erik. "River Blindness: Conquering an Ancient Scourge." *New York Times*, January 8, 1989. http://www.nytimes.com/1989/01/08/magazine
/river-blindness-conquering-an-ancient-scourge.html?pagewanted=all.

Ekwunife, Chinyelu Angela. "Socio-Economic and Water Contact Studies in *Schistosomiasis haematobium* Infested Area of Anambra State, Nigeria." *Animal Research International* 1(3) (2004): 200–202. https://www.zoo-unn
.org/index.php/ARI/article/view/448.

Ekwunife, Chinyelu A., Fabian C. Okafor, and Obioma C. Mwaorgu. "Ultrasonic Screening of Urinary Schistosomiasis Infected Patients in Agulu Community, Anambra State, Southeast Nigeria." *International Archives of Medicine* 2 (2009). doi:10.1186/1755-7682-2-34.

Fan, Kawai, and Honkei Lai. "Mao Zedong's Fight against Schistosomiasis." *Perspectives in Biology and Medicine* 51(2) (2008): 176–87. https://muse.jhu
.edu/article/236273.

Farley, John. *To Cast Out Disease: A History of the International Health Division of the Rockefeller Foundation (1913–1951).* New York: Oxford University Press, 2004.

Fitzpatrick, Christopher, et al. "An Investment Case for Ending Neglected Tropical Diseases." In *Major Infectious Diseases*, vol. 6 of *Disease Control Priorities*, 3rd ed., edited by King K. Holmes et al., 411–32. Washington,

DC: World Bank. http://dcp-3.org/chapter/2377/investment-case-ending
-neglected-tropical-diseases.

Fleming, David. "Neglected No More: Ending Neglected Tropical Diseases
Helps Us All." *Huffington Post*, March 20, 2017. http://www.huffington
post.com/entry/neglect-no-more-ending-neglected-tropical-diseases_us
_58d011aee4b0537abd95734e.

Flora, Victor, and Anthony Solomon. "Neglected No More: Ending Trachoma, an Infectious Eye Disease Rooted in Poverty." *Guardian*, April 24,
2017. https://www.theguardian.com/global-development-professionals
-network/2017/apr/24/visionary-approach-saving-millions-trachoma.

Foege, William H. *House on Fire: The Fight to Eradicate Smallpox*. Berkeley:
University of California Press, 2011.

Garba, Amadou, et al. "Implementation of National Schistosomiasis Control
Programmes in West Africa." *Trends in Parasitology* 22(7) (2006): 322-26.
doi:10.1016/j.pt.2006.04.007.

Gates, Bill. "Here's My Plan to Improve Our World—And How You Can
Help." *Wired*, November 12, 2013. https://www.wired.com/2013/11/bill
-gates-wired-essay.

Gates Foundation. "Grant of $30 Million to Establish the Schistosomiasis
Control Initiative to Give Hope to Developing Countries." 2002. www
.gatesfoundation.org/Media-Center/Press-Releases/2002/07/%20Schisto
somiasis-Control-Initiative-Receives-Grant.

Geneva Global. "Rwanda and Burundi Tropical Disease Control: 2007–2010
Report." March 2011. In possession of author.

Gibbs, W. Wayt. "Bill Gates Views Good Data as Key to Global Health." *Scientific American*, August 1, 2016. https://www.scientificamerican.com
/article/bill-gates-interview-good-data-key-to-global-health.

Hall, Andrew, and Sue Horton. "Deworming." 2009. http://www.copen
hagenconsensus.com/sites/default/files/deworming.pdf.

Hall, Andrew, Yaobi Zhang, et al. "The Role of Nutrition in Integrated Programs to Control Neglected Tropical Diseases." *BMC Medicine* 10 (2012):
41. http://www.biomedcentral.com/1741-7015/10/41.

Hanke, Steve H., and Alex K. F. Kwok. "On the Measurement of Zimbabwe's
Hyperinflation." *Cato Journal* 29(2) (Spring/Summer 2009): 353-64.

Horton, Sue, Harold Alderman, and Juan A. Rivera. "The Challenge of Hunger and Malnutrition." In *Global Crises, Global Solutions*, edited by Bjørn
Lomborg, 305-33. Cambridge: Cambridge University Press, 2009.

Hotez, Peter J. *Blue Marble Health: An Innovative Plan to Fight Diseases of the Poor amid Wealth*. Baltimore, MD: Johns Hopkins University Press, 2016.

———. *Forgotten People, Forgotten Diseases: The Neglected Tropical Diseases and Their Impact on Global Health and Development*. Washington, DC: AMS Press, 2013.

Hotez, Peter J., and Aruna Kamath. "Neglected Tropical Diseases in Sub-Saharan Africa: Review of Their Prevalence, Distribution, and Disease Burden." *PLOS Neglected Tropical Diseases* 3 (2009): e412. doi:10.1371/jour nal.pntd.0000412.

Hotez, Peter J., David H. Molyneux, et al. "Control of Neglected Tropical Diseases." *New England Journal of Medicine* 357 (2007): 1018–27.

International Coalition for Trachoma Control. "The End in Sight: 2020 INSight." July 2011. http://www.trachomacoalition.org/sites/default /files/content/resources/files/ICTC_EnglishJuly21lowres.pdf.

Jack, Andrew. "Gates Finds Controversy Even in Works of Charity." *Financial Times*, June 12, 2006. https://www.ft.com/content/aa076b9e-fa40 -11da-b7ff-0000779e2340?mhq5j=e1.

———. "The Long Road to Elimination of Neglected Tropical Diseases." *Financial Times*, April 18, 2017. https://www.ft.com/content/a7904aae-0266 -11e7-aa5b-6bb07f5c8e12.

Kabatereine, Narcis B., et al. "How to (or Not to) Integrate Vertical Programmes for the Control of Major Neglected Tropical Diseases in Sub-Saharan Africa." *PLOS Neglected Tropical Diseases* 4 (2010): e755. doi:10.1371/journal.pntd.0000755.

Keating, Conrad. *Kenneth Warren and the Great Neglected Diseases of Mankind Programme: The Transformation of Geographical Medicine in the US and Beyond*. Oxford: Springer, 2017.

Kierman, Frank A., Jr. "The Blood Fluke That Saved Formosa." *Harper's Magazine*, April 1959. https://harpers.org/archive/1959/04/the-blood-fluke-that -saved-formosa.

Kirsch, Vanessa, Jim Bildner, and Jeff Walker. "Why Social Ventures Need Systems Thinking." *Harvard Business Review*, July 25, 2016. https://hbr .org/2016/07/why-social-ventures-need-systems-thinking.

Krauth, Stefanie J., et al. "An In-Depth Analysis of a Piece of Shit: Distribution of *Schistosoma mansoni* and Hookworm Eggs in Human Stool." *PLOS Neglected Tropical Diseases* 6 (2012): e1969. doi:10.1371/journal .pntd.0001969.

Lammie, Patrick J., et al. "Translating Research into Reality: Elimination of Lymphatic Filariasis from Haiti." *American Journal of Tropical Medicine and Hygiene* 97 (October 2017): 71-75. doi:10.4269/ajtmh.16-0669.

Levine, Ruth, and the What Works Working Group with Molly Kinder. *Millions Saved: Proven Successes in Global Health.* Washington, DC: Center for Global Development, 2004.

Liese, Bernard H., et al. *The Onchocerciasis Control Program in West Africa: A Long-Term Commitment to Success.* Washington, DC: World Bank, August 1991.

Litt, Elizabeth, Margaret C. Baker, and David Molyneux. "Neglected Tropical Diseases and Mental Health: A Perspective on Comorbidity." *Trends in Parasitology* 28 (2012): 195-201. doi:10.1016/j.pt.2012.03.001.

Lo, Nathan C., et al. "Comparison of Community-Wide, Integrated Mass Drug Administration Strategies for Schistosomiasis and Soil-Transmitted Helminthiasis: A Cost-Effectiveness Modelling Study." *Lancet* 3 (2015): e629-38. doi:10.1016/S2214-109X(15)00047-9.

MacAskill, William. *Doing Good Better: How Effective Altruism Can Help Make a Difference.* New York: Gotham, 2015.

McGuire, Robert A., and Philip R. P. Coelho. *Parasites, Pathogens, and Progress: Diseases and Economic Development.* Cambridge, MA: MIT Press, 2011.

"Merck Offers Free Distribution of New River Blindness Drug." *New York Times*, October 22, 1987. http://www.nytimes.com/1987/10/22/world /merck-offers-free-distribution-of-new-river-blindness-drug.html.

Miguel, Edward, and Michael Kremer. "Worms: Identifying Impacts on Education and Health in the Presence of Treatment Externalities." *Econometrica* 72 (2004): 159-217. http://cega.berkeley.edu/assets/cega_research _projects/1/Identifying-Impacts-on-Education-and-Health-in-the-Presence -of-Treatment-Externalities.pdf.

Molyneux, David H. "Combating the 'Other Diseases' of MDG 6: Changing the Paradigm to Achieve Equity and Poverty Reduction?" *Transactions of the Royal Society of Tropical Medicine and Hygiene* 102 (2008): 509-19. doi:10.1016/j.trstmh.2008.02.024.

———. "'Neglected' Diseases but Unrecognised Successes: Challenges and Opportunities for Infectious Disease Control." *Lancet* 364 (2004). http:// image.thelancet.com/extras/03art7073web.pdf.

Molyneux, David H., and Steve A. Ward. "Reflections on the Nobel Prize for

Medicine 2015: The Public Health Legacy and Impact of Avermectin and Artemisinin." *Trends in Parasitology* 31 (2015): 605–7.

Moses, Sue-Lynn. "Neglected No More? The Fight against NTDs Picks Up." *Inside Philanthropy*, April 20, 2017. https://www.insidephilanthropy.com /home/2017/4/20/neglected-no-more-the-fight-against-ntds-just-got-much -bigger.

Musgrove, Philip, and Peter J. Hotez. "Turning Neglected Tropical Diseases into Forgotten Maladies." *Health Affairs* 28 (2009): 1691–706. doi:10.1377 /hlthaff.28.6.1691.

Mwandawiro, Charles S., et al. "Monitoring and Evaluating the Impact of National School-Based Deworming in Kenya: Study Design and Baseline Results." *Parasites and Vectors* 6 (2013). https://doi.org/10.1186/1756-3305 -6-198.

Newbury, David S. *Kings and Clans: Idjwi Island and the Lake Kivu Rift, 1780–1840*. Madison: University of Wisconsin Press, 1991.

Norris, Jeremiah, et al. *Social and Economic Impact Review on Neglected Tropical Diseases*. Washington, DC: Hudson Institute, 2012.

Ohenjo, Nyang'ori, et al. "Health of Indigenous People in Africa." *Lancet* 367 (2006): 1937–46. http://dx.doi.org/10.1016/S0140-6736(06)68849-1.

Ozier, Owen. *Exploiting Externalities to Estimate the Long-Term Effects of Early Childhood Deworming*. Washington, DC: World Bank Development Group, February 22, 2017.

Redekop, William K., et al. "The Socioeconomic Benefit to Individuals of Achieving the 2020 Targets for Five Preventive Chemotherapy Neglected Tropical Diseases." *PLOS Neglected Tropical Diseases* 11 (2017): e0005289. https://doi.org/10.1371/journal.pntd.0005289.

Republic of Rwanda Ministry of Health and Rwanda Biomedical Center. "Mapping of Schistosomiasis and Soil-Transmitted Helminthiasis in Rwanda 2014: Mapping Survey Report." February 2015. In possession of author.

Rockefeller Foundation. *Shared Journey: The Rockefeller Foundation, Human Capital, and Development in Africa*. New York: Rockefeller Foundation, 2013.

Rodger, F. C. *Blindness in West Africa*. London: Royal Commonwealth Society for the Blind, 1959.

Rotondo, Lisa A., et al. "The Neglected Tropical Disease Non-Governmental Development Organization Network (NNN): The Value and Future of a

Global Network Aiming to Control and Eliminate NTDs." *International Health* 8 (2016): i4–i6. doi:10.1093/inthealth/ihw004.

Ruxin, Josh, and Joel Negin. "Removing the Neglect from Neglected Tropical Diseases: The Rwandan Experience, 2008–2010." *Global Public Health* 7 (2012): 812–22. http://dx.doi.org/10.1080/17441692.2012.699535.

Schlosser, Katherine. "History of Trachoma." *International Trachoma Initiative*, n.d. http://www.trachomacoalition.org/sites/default/files/content /resources/files/History%20of%20Trachoma%20by%20Katherine%20 Schlosser.pdf.

"Secrets of Sovereign." *Institutional Investor*, March 16, 2006. http://www .institutionalinvestor.com/article/1019610/secrets-of-sovereign.html# .WYDSB9MrJAY.

Sheshadri, Raja. "Pygmies in the Congo Basin and Conflict." *ICE Case Studies* 163 (2005). http://mandalaprojects.com/ice/ice-cases/pygmy.htm.

Shin, Ji-Hye. "The 'Oriental' Problem: Trachoma and Asian Immigrants in the United States, 1897–1910." *Korean Journal of Medical History* 23 (2014): 573–606. doi:10.13081/kjmh.2014.23.573.

Singer, Peter. *The Life You Can Save: Acting Now to End World Poverty.* New York: Random House, 2009.

Smith, James, and Emma Michelle Taylor. "MDGs and NTDs: Reshaping the Global Health Agenda." *PLOS Neglected Tropical Diseases* 7 (2013): e2529. doi:10.1371/journal.pntd.0002529.

Stenberg, Karin, et al. "Financing Transformative Health Systems towards Achievement of the Health Sustainable Development Goals: A Model for Projected Resource Needs in 67 Low-Income and Middle-Income Countries." *Lancet* 5(9) (2017). http://dx.doi.org/10.1016/S2214-109X(17)30263-2.

Stepan, Nancy Leys. *Eradication: Ridding the World of Diseases Forever?* Ithaca, NY: Cornell University Press, 2011.

Stoll, Norman R. "This Wormy World." *Journal of Parasitology* 33 (1947): 1–18. http://www.jstor.org/stable/3273613.

Tapureta, Beaven. "Young Writers Show Africa the Way." *Herald* (Zimbabwe), July 6, 2016. http://www.herald.co.zw/young-writers-show-africa-the-way.

Useem, Michael. "Roy Vagelos Attacks River Blindness." In Useem, *The Leadership Moment: Nine True Stories of Triumph and Disaster and Their Lessons for Us All*, 10–42. New York: Three Rivers Press, 1998.

Vagelos, Roy, and Louis Galambos. *Medicine, Science, and Merck.* New York: Cambridge University Press, 2004.

Walker, Jeffrey C. "Solving the World's Biggest Problems: Better Philan-
    thropy through Systems Change." *Stanford Social Innovation Review*, April
    5, 2017. https://ssir.org/articles/entry/solving_the_worlds_biggest_prob
    lems_better_philanthropy_through_systems_cha.
Warren, Kenneth S., et al. "Helminth Infection." In *Disease Control Priorities
    in Developing Countries*, edited by D. T. Jamison et al., 131-60. Oxford:
    Oxford University Press, 1993.
Webster, Joanne P., et al. "The Contribution of Mass Drug Administration to
    Global Health: Past, Present and Future." *Philosophical Transactions of the
    Royal Society B* 369 (2014). http://dx.doi.org/10.1098/rstb.2013.0434.
Welch, Vivian A., et al. "Deworming and Adjuvant Interventions for Improv-
    ing the Developmental Health and Well-Being of Children in Low- and
    Middle-Income Countries: A Systematic Review and Network Meta-
    Analysis." *Campbell Systematic Reviews* (2016). https://www.campbellcol
    laboration.org/library/mass-deworming-interventions-child-health.html.
West, Sheila K. "Azithromycin for Control of Trachoma." *Community Eye
    Health* 12 (1999): 55-56. https://www.ncbi.nlm.nih.gov/pmc/articles
    /PMC1706032/pdf/jceh_12_32_055.pdf.
Wilson, John. *Travelling Blind*. 1963. Reprint. London: Adventurers Club,
    1964.
World Bank. *Investing in Health: World Development Report 1993*. New York:
    Oxford University Press, 1993.
World Health Organization. *Accelerating Work to Overcome the Global Impact
    of Neglected Tropical Diseases: A Roadmap for Implementation*. Geneva:
    World Health Organization, 2012.
———. *Future Approaches to Trachoma Control: Report of a Global Scientific Meet-
    ing*. Geneva: World Health Organization, 1997.
———. *Report of the Tenth Meeting of the WHO Strategic and Technical Advisory
    Group for Neglected Tropical Diseases*. Geneva: World Health Organiza-
    tion, March 29-30, 2017. http://www.who.int/neglected_diseases/NTD
    _STAG_report_2017.pdf?ua=1.
———. *Weekly Epidemiological Report* 89(39) (September 26, 2014): 421-28.
    http://www.who.int/wer/2013/wer8939.pdf.
Zhang, Yaobi, et al. "Control of Neglected Tropical Diseases Needs a Long-
    Term Commitment." *BMC Medicine* 8 (2010). https://doi.org/10.1186/1741
    -7015-8-67.
Zimbabwe Ministry of Health and Child Welfare. "National Strategic

Plan and Programme for the Control of Neglected Tropical Diseases,
2012-2016." N.d. In possession of author.

———. "Training Manual, 2012-2016: Mass Drug Administration (MDA) for
Schistosomiasis (Bilharzia) and Soil Transmitted Helminths (Intestinal
Worms)." N.d. In possession of author.

Zimmer, Carl. *Parasite Rex: Inside the Bizarre World of Nature's Most Dangerous
Creatures*. New York: Free Press, 2000.

INDEX